SCALING UP ONE HEALTH APPROACHES IN THE GREATER MEKONG SUBREGION

NOVEMBER 2024

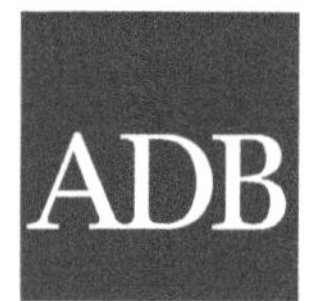

ASIAN DEVELOPMENT BANK

CONTENTS

TABLES, FIGURES, AND BOXES

ACKNOWLEDGMENTS

This report was authored by Rikard Elfving, a principal social sector specialist at the Asian Development Bank (ADB); Jane Parry, a consultant health and development analyst; and Eric Neumann, a veterinary epidemiology and livestock health consultant.

From ADB, the authors would like to thank Srinivasan Ancha, Ben Coghlan, Najibullah Habib, and Natasha Kuruppu. The authors would also like to thank Nansubuga Isdahl, consultant with ADB's Health Practice team in the Sectors Group for her invaluable feedback, comments, and edits.

From the Nossal Institute for Global Health, the authors would like to thank Angus Campbell, Clare Strachan, Max Barot, Xuefeng Zhong, Melanie Bannister-Tyrrell, Krishna Hort, Ajay Mahal, Barbara McPake, Anna Barrett, Mark Stevenson, and Divya Sama.

The authors are grateful for the invaluable contributions of Greater Mekong Subregion partners and key development partners.

ABBREVIATIONS

ADB	Asian Development Bank
AMR	Antimicrobial resistance
APHSAF	Asia Pacific Health Security Action Framework
ASEAN	Association of Southeast Asian Nations
PRC	People's Republic of China
COVID-19	coronavirus disease (COVID-19)
FAO	Food and Agriculture Organization of the United Nations
GMS	Greater Mekong Subregion
IHR	International Health Regulations
OHP	One Health Partnership
Lao PDR	Lao People's Democratic Republic
RCZI	Roadmap to Combat Zoonoses in India
SARS	severe acute respiratory syndrome
SASEC	South Asia Subregional Economic Cooperation
SEAOHUN	Southeast Asia One Health University Network
SEARO	South-East Asia Regional Office
TA	technical assistance
UN	United Nations
UNEP	United Nations Environment Programme
USAID	United States Agency for International Development
WHO	World Health Organization
WOAH	World Organisation for Animal Health

EXECUTIVE SUMMARY

Climate change is the single biggest threat to human health due to increased air pollution, extreme weather events, and forced displacement. It is also exacerbating other dangers, including food security and safety, antimicrobial resistance (AMR) whereby bacteria, viruses, fungi, and parasites change over time and stop responding to medicines, and human vulnerability to diseases of animal origin, or zoonoses. The novel coronavirus (COVID-19) that led to a pandemic with devastating economic and social consequences in Asia and the Pacific is unlikely to be the last pandemic of its kind. These global phenomena are also playing out in the Greater Mekong Subregion (GMS), which has been identified as a hot spot for emerging zoonotic diseases, as well as AMR.

The health impact of climate change poses such a significant threat to economic development that it cannot be successfully addressed by one sector alone. One Health, an integrated, unifying approach that aims to sustainably balance and optimize the health of people, animals, and ecosystems. It is a powerful approach to help conceptualize crosscutting initiatives and to address opportunities and challenges related to One Health. In the post-COVID-19 era, and in anticipation of possible future pandemics, the One Health approach is a way of building multisectoral alliances that can better protect regional health security. One Health processes are the ways in which this concept can be put into practice.

This publication provides an overview of One Health in the GMS and its relationship to addressing climate change there. It details One Health activities in the subregion and recommends how they can be scaled up, including specific investment opportunities. These recommendations are derived from detailed country consultations and communication with ministries of agriculture, environment, and health in the GMS.

GMS countries have already made explicit commitments to adopting a One Health approach. Under the GMS Economic Cooperation Program Strategic Framework 2030, every GMS country already has some multisector One Health information-sharing mechanism. Most also have joint surveillance and response capacity. However, there are many gaps in resources (including infrastructure, human resources, and institutional capacity). Engagement on One Health with the private sector, subnational levels of government, civil society, and communities has been suboptimal.

In the GMS context, many One Health interventions are already achievable to tackle specific issues. Examples include investing in policy, legislation, and regulation of wildlife use in the GMS; integrating wildlife surveillance into national One Health surveillance systems in the GMS countries; building the capacity of the workforce in the animal health and environment sectors; and investing in climate change-focused and disease-specific initiatives.

Because One Health actions are complex and cut across multiple sectors, they call for extra coordination among development partners and within governments. Joint action and coordination among key development partners is critical to successful One Health programming. This applies to partners with a diverse range of mandates, including human and animal health, environmental protection, gender, development finance, and climate change.

This paper can be used as guidance for scaling up and improving One Health work in the GMS, in line with the new GMS Health Cooperation Strategy 2024–2030, the upcoming revision of the Asia Pacific Strategy for Emerging Diseases, and other major milestone global initiatives on climate change and One Health. The key action areas for GMS countries to increase their use of the One Health framework also align with the priority actions of the United Nations One Health Quadripartite-led global call to action for One Health for a safer world.

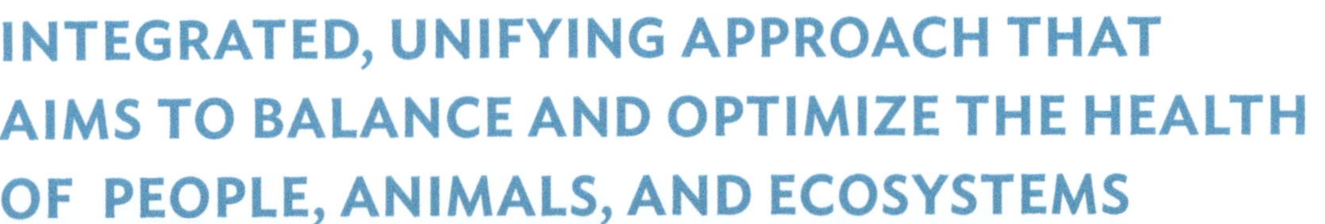

INTEGRATED, UNIFYING APPROACH THAT
AIMS TO BALANCE AND OPTIMIZE THE HEALTH
OF PEOPLE, ANIMALS, AND ECOSYSTEMS

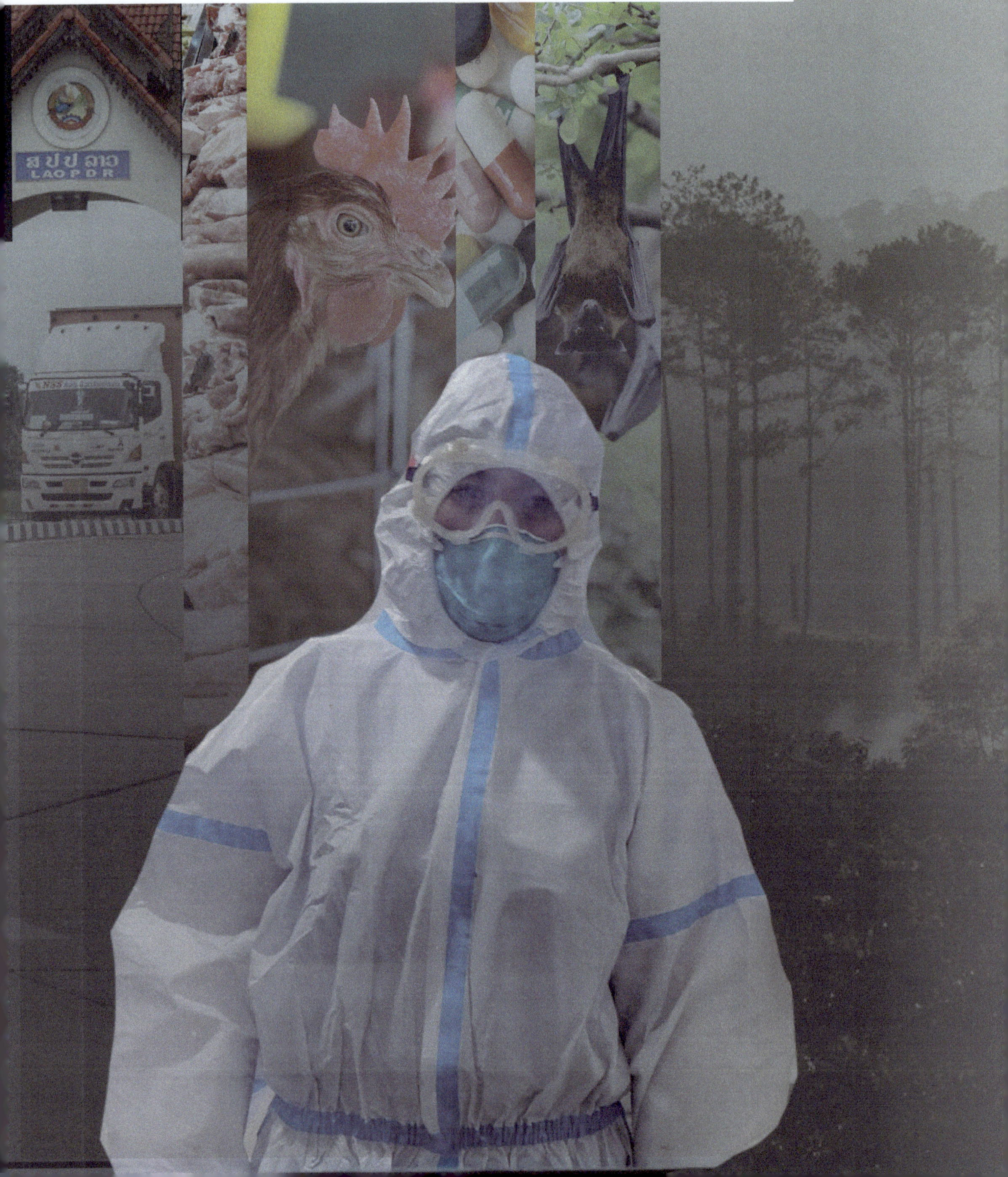

PREVENT AND REDUCE IMPACT OF **CLIMATE CHANGE**

IDENTIFY AND PRESERVE CARBON STORING ECOSYSTEMS

ADOPT TECHNOLOGIES TO REDUCE OR RECLAIM CARBON EMISSIONS

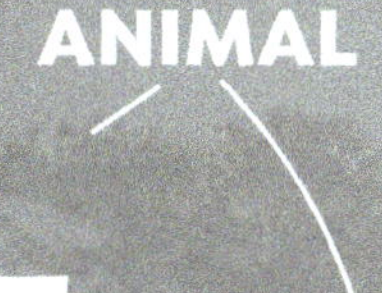

BUILD RESILIENCE TO DISEASE RISK

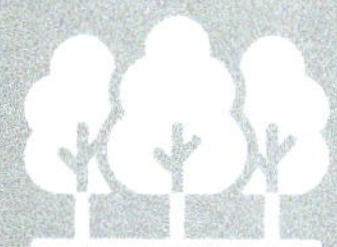

INVEST IN NATURE BASED SOLUTIONS

ENHANCE FOOD SECURITY

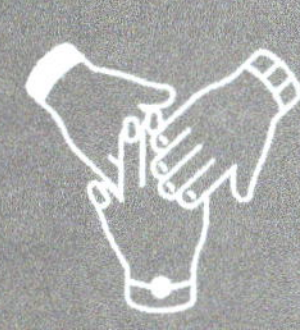

FOSTER CROSSCUTTING INITIATIVES

HELP MAKE INFORMED DECISION

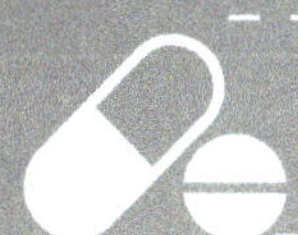

PREVENT EXCESS DEATH DUE TO ANTIMICROBIAL RESISTANCE

GREATER MEKONG SUBREGION

Countries are scaling up their commitments to One Health approach

WHAT'S HAPPENING ALREADY

- ☑ Multisector One Health information-sharing mechanism
- ☑ Joint surveillance and response capacity

WHAT STILL NEEDS TO HAPPEN

- ☐ Engagement on One Health with the private sector, subnational government, civil society, and communities
- ☐ Filling gaps in resources including infrastructure, human resources, and institutional capacity
- ☐ Policy, legislation, and regulation of wildlife use, and integrate wildlife surveillance into One Health

ONE HEALTH— ADDRESSING CLIMATE AND HEALTH RISKS IN THE GREATER MEKONG SUBREGION

Both climate change and the coronavirus disease (COVID-19) pandemic have brought renewed attention to the interconnectedness of health challenges and the need for multisector approaches to reduce and respond to complex health threats. Climate change is the single biggest threat to human health.[1] It is directly connected to environmental pollution and threats to biodiversity and wildlife habitats, as well as human health.[2] Climate change is worsening food security and safety, and antimicrobial resistance (AMR), whereby bacteria, viruses, fungi and parasites change over time and stop responding to medicines.[3] At the same time, human vulnerability to diseases of animal origin, or zoonoses, is also on the rise, and is exacerbated by environmental factors.[4] As an example of a recent zoonosis, the novel coronavirus disease (COVID-19) led to a pandemic with devastating economic and social consequences in Asia and the Pacific.[5] COVID-19 is unlikely to be the last pandemic of its kind: an estimated three out of four new infectious disease outbreaks are zoonoses. (Footnote 3) Moreover, novel viral outbreaks are occurring with increasing frequency.[6]

The Greater Mekong Subregion (GMS)[7] has been identified as a hot spot for emerging zoonotic diseases.[8] It is characterized by rapid agricultural and urban development, deforestation, and the formal and informal transboundary movement of people and animals. These factors are all associated with emergence of zoonoses.[9] In the GMS, like the rest of Asia and the Pacific, zoonoses have adverse effects on livelihoods and trade as well as health.[10] Pandemics are costly: the COVID-19 pandemic caused a 4.4% contraction in the global economy in 2020.[11] Previous disease outbreaks, such as the 2003 severe acute respiratory syndrome (SARS) epidemic, have also taken an economic toll. The Asian Development Bank (ADB) estimated the economic impact of SARS as

---

1   United Nations. Climate Action Fast Facts.
2   Zhang, R., Tang, X., Liu, J., et al. 2022. From concept to action: a united, holistic and One Health approach to respond to the climate change crisis. *Infect Dis Poverty.* 11(17).
3   World Health Organization. Antimicrobial resistance.
4   US Centers for Disease Control and Prevention. Zoonotic Diseases.
5   Asian Development Bank. 2023. *Annual Report 2022.*
6   Bernstein A.S., et al. 2022. The costs and benefits of primary prevention of zoonotic pandemics. *Sciences Advances.* 8. eab14183.
7   Cambodia, Lao People's Democratic Republic, Myanmar, Thailand, Viet Nam, and People's Republic of China.
8   Allen, T. et al. 2017. Global hotspots and correlates of emerging zoonotic diseases. *Nature Communications.* 8. p. 1124.
9   Berthe,F. C. J., Bali, S., R., and Batmanian, G. J. 2022. *Putting Pandemics Behind Us: Investing in One Health to Reduce Risks of Emerging Infectious Diseases* (English). World Bank Group.
10 Shrestha, S. 2019. What Asia Can Do to Protect against Animal-Borne Diseases. *Development Asia.* Manila: Asian Development Bank. 30 August.
11 Markotter, W., et al. One Health High-Level Export Panel. Prevention of Zoonotic Spillover. From Relying on Response to Reducing the Risk at Source. One Health High-Level Export Panel.

approximately $18 billion in East Asia, or around 0.6% of gross domestic product.[12]

For GMS countries, the threat of pandemics is further compounded by other climate-related challenges, including AMR, and pressure on food security and safety. The impact on health of all these factors poses such a significant threat to economic development in the GMS that it cannot be successfully addressed by one sector alone.

One Health: A Framework for an Interdependent World

One Health is an approach to human, animal, plant, and ecological health challenges that starts from a simple premise: these are all interconnected, and their solution demands communication, coordination, and collaboration across multiple sectors, disciplines, and levels of government.[13] Its aspirations are a healthy ecosystem, healthy community, and healthy people with sustainable livelihoods.[14]

The essence of One Health is interdependence (Figure 1), and this is what makes the One Health framework especially powerful for conceptualizing crosscutting initiatives and helping people break down siloed thinking and work practices. One Health processes are the ways in which this concept can be put into practice. In the post-COVID-19 era, and in anticipation of possible future pandemics, the One Health approach is a way of building multisectoral alliances that can better protect regional health security. However, it is also precisely this lack of

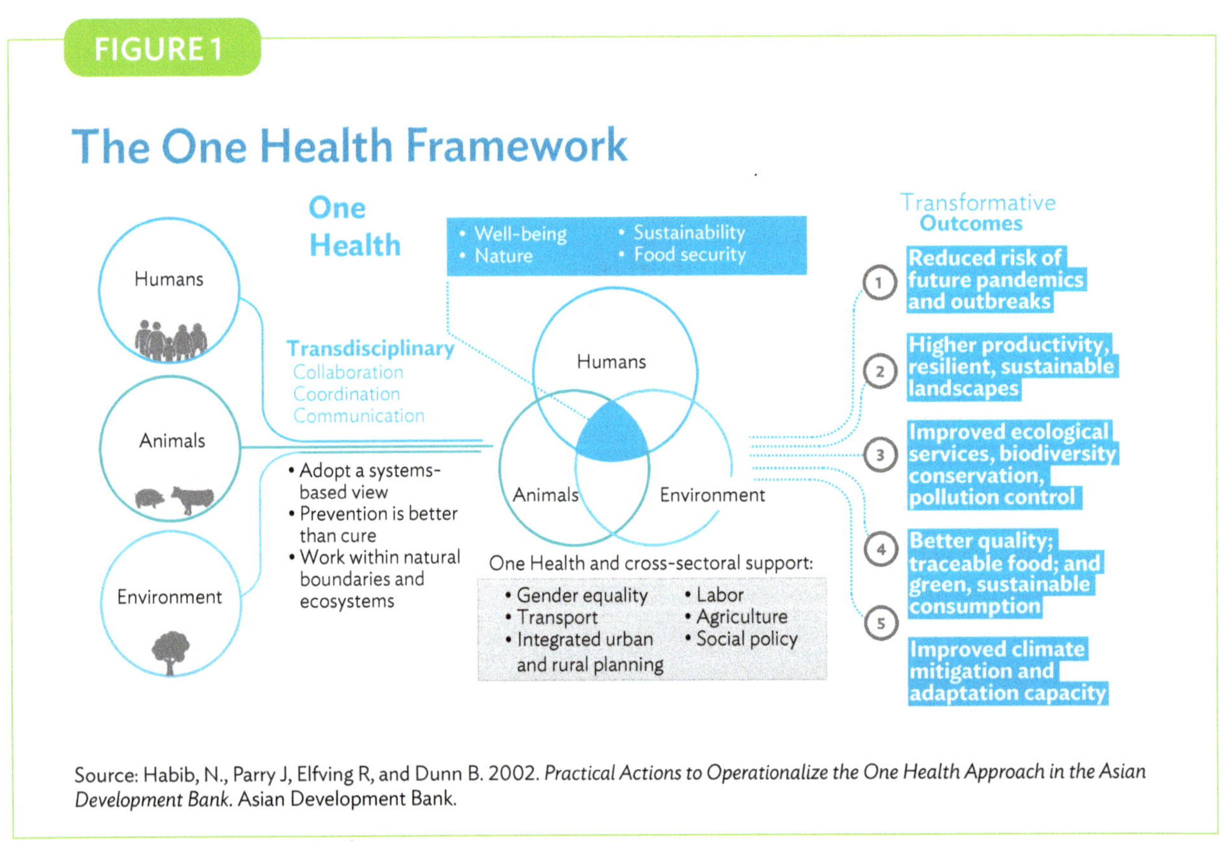

Source: Habib, N., Parry J, Elfving R, and Dunn B. 2002. *Practical Actions to Operationalize the One Health Approach in the Asian Development Bank.* Asian Development Bank.

---

12 Fan, E. 2003. SARS: Economic Impact and Implications. *ERD Policy Brief.* No. 15. Manila: Economic Research and Development Impact Department, Asian Development Bank.

13 Food and Agriculture Organization, World Organisation for Animal Health, UN Environment Programme, World Health Organization. 2021. *One Health High-Level Expert Panel Annual Report 2021.*

14 Evans, B.R., and F.A. Leighton. 2014. A History of One Health. *Rev. Sci. Tech. Off. Int. Epiz.* 33 (2). pp. 413–420.

single-issue focus that makes adopting a One Health approach challenging—it often means that there is a lack of strong coordination and strong governance structure at both national and regional levels.

One Health relates to almost every one of the Sustainable Development Goals (SDGs). The Lancet One Health Commission notes that the SDGs "in themselves can be understood as embodying a One Health strategy aimed at healthy people living on a perpetually habitable planet."[15] Because One Health approaches can be applied from the international through regional, national, subnational and community levels, they support change at all levels, from governance to grassroots initiatives.

Globally, four agencies have taken the lead on One Health. The United Nations One Health Quadripartite consists of the Food and Agriculture Organization of the United Nations (FAO), United Nations Environment Programme (UNEP), World Health Organization (WHO) and World Organisation for Animal Health (WOAH). In 2022, the Quadripartite published its *One Health Joint Plan of Action (2022–2026): Working Together for the Health of Humans, Animals, Plants and the Environment.*[16] The plan promotes multisectoral collaboration to expand One Health capacities along six action tracks (Figure 2). These action tracks point to opportunities for other development partners, such as ADB, to help countries scale up One Health actions. The One Health framework also aligns with numerous health security initiatives (Box 1), and with the aims of the Pandemic Fund (Box 2).

The One Health Quadripartite Joint Plan of Action Tracks

Source: Food and Agriculture Organization of the United Nations, United Nations Environment Programme, World Health Organization and World Organisation for Animal Health. 2022. *Global Plan of Action on One Health. Towards a More Comprehensive One Health Approach to Global Health Threats at the Human-Animal-Environment Interface.* Rome.

[15]   Amuasi, J. H., et al. 2020. Reconnecting for Our Future: The Lancet One Health Commission. *The Lancet.* 395(10235). pp. 1469–1471.
[16]   Food and Agriculture Organization of the United Nations, UN Environment Programme, World Health Organization, World Organisation for Animal Health. 2022. One Health Joint Plan of Action (2022–2026). Working Together for the Health of Humans, Animals, Plants and the Environment.

BOX 1

One Health and Health Security Initiatives

The 2005 International Health Regulations (IHR) were agreed upon by World Health Organization (WHO) member states, as a set of rights and obligations for countries, including the requirement to report public health events. The WHO Joint External Evaluation (JEE) tool is the mechanism by which countries can assess their preparedness for compliance with implementation of the IHR. The original IHR were a response to the 2003 SARS epidemic, have been amended twice (in 2014 and 2022), and are being amended again, in the wake of the coronavirus disease (COVID-19) pandemic after consultations with member states. The most recent amendments came into effect on 1 June 2024.[a] One Health is incorporated in all components of the IHR Monitoring and Evaluation Framework.

The Asia Pacific Health Security Action Framework (APHSAF), currently under development, builds on the strong foundations of the Asia Pacific Strategy for Emerging Diseases and Public Health Emergencies (APSED), which was last updated in 2016, and was designed to support the reduction of the health risks and consequences from emergencies at the community, subnational, national, regional, and global levels by developing, strengthening, and improving health security and health systems resilience through implementation of the IHR.[b]

Whereas APSED had eight focus areas, the APHSAF takes an interconnected "domain" approach to health security, and emphasizes multisectoral, whole-of-society and whole-of-government engagement in comprehensive health security. In particular, the leadership domain emphasizes the need for cooperation across sectors and between countries, which is entirely in line with One Health's emphasis on communication, coordination, collaboration, and integration.

APHSAF is based on these core values: equity; leaving no one behind; inclusivity; engaging all stakeholders in leadership and decision-making; coherence; and connecting health security systems and initiatives at the subnational, national, regional, and global levels. It emphasizes multisectoral collaboration and coordination within and beyond the health sector. In May 2023, the Association of Southeast Asian Nations (ASEAN) leaders' One Health Initiative Declaration committed to establishing the ASEAN One Health Network to promote multisectoral collaboration and coordination of One Health initiatives among member states. ASEAN also pledged to develop a One Health Joint Plan of Action to improve regional and national capacity and capabilities with targets that are tangible, measurable, and time-bound, including through bilateral and multilateral cooperation; and to encourage ASEAN member states to consolidate all One Health initiatives and mainstream the approach.[c]

Asia Pacific Health Security Action Framework Domains

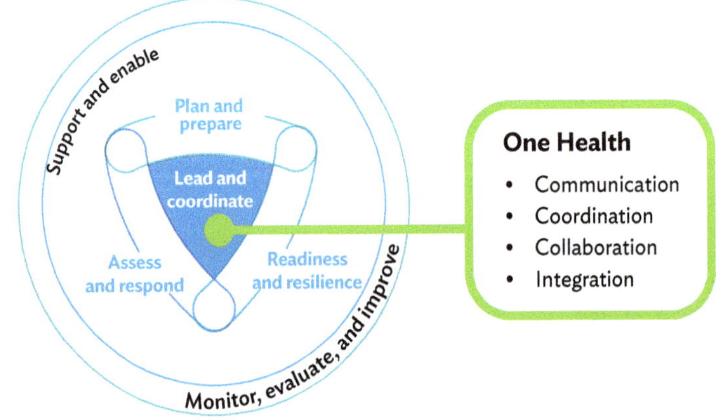

Source: WHO.

[a] World Health Organization. 2023. Governments make progress towards agreeing amendments to the International Health Regulations. Geneva. 7 October.
[b] Presentation by Qiu Yi Khut, technical officer, Public Health Emergency Preparedness WHO Health Emergencies Programme. WHO Regional Office for the Western Pacific. 13 December 2023.
[c] ASEAN. 2023. ASEAN Leaders' Declaration on One Health Initiative.

BOX 2

The Pandemic Fund and One Health

The multistakeholder global partnership, the Pandemic Fund, hosted by the World Bank, provides a dedicated stream of additional, long-term financing to strengthen pandemic prevention, preparedness, and response capacity and capabilities in low- and middle-income countries.[a] The Pandemic Fund's objectives are to bring additional, dedicated resources for pandemic prevention, preparedness, and response; to incentivize countries to increase investments in One Health; to enhance coordination among partners; and to serve as a platform for advocacy.

In 2023, the Pandemic Fund awarded a total of $338 million in grants that will mobilize over $2 billion of co-funding from governments and donor organizations to help 37 countries strengthen their capacity to prevent, prepare for, and respond to pandemics. Within the Greater Mekong Subregion, the Cambodia Pandemic Prevention, Preparedness, and Response project submitted by the Kingdom of Cambodia and with World Bank, the Food and Agriculture Organization of the United Nations, and Asian Infrastructure Investment Bank acting as implementing entities, was one of the funded projects.

The Pandemic Fund's second round of funding in 2024, worth $500 million will be followed by two further rounds of funding likely being launched in 2024–2025, subject to available resources. The second funding round call for proposals continues to prioritize high-impact investments in early warning and disease surveillance systems, laboratory systems, and human resources for health, and community workforce capacity strengthening, related to human and animal health. All six GMS countries are eligible to seek funding from the Pandemic Fund, either individually or as part of a regional project. Project implementation must involve one or more of the Fund's 13 approved implementing entities, which include the Asian Development Bank.

[a] World Bank. FAQs: 2022. The Pandemic Fund. 30 June.

One Health and Climate Change in the Greater Mekong Subregion

Climate change is forcing a radical rethink of humanity's relationship with other species and the environment. Due to effects of climate change, the Asia and Pacific region is at extreme risk of undoing the economic and social development gains realized over recent years (Figure 3).[17] Climate change carries a significant cost to human health. For example, modeling shows that climate change is expected to cause 250,000 additional deaths per year between 2030 and 2050 globally, including 144,000 deaths due to viral diarrhea and malaria, and 95,000 attributable to childhood undernutrition.[18] Climate change is leading to increased health security risks around the world, including in the GMS.

One Health offers a framework to address these risks and engage in both climate change adaptation and resilience and supports the fulfillment of global and regional climate change commitments (Box 3).

---

[17]   Asian Development Bank. 2021. *Disaster Resilience in Asia—A Special Supplement of Asia's Journey to Prosperity: Policy, Market, and Technology Over 50 Years.* Manila.
[18]   World Health Organization. 2018. *COP24 Special Report: Health & Climate Change.* Poland.

FIGURE 3

The Climate Change–One Health Nexus

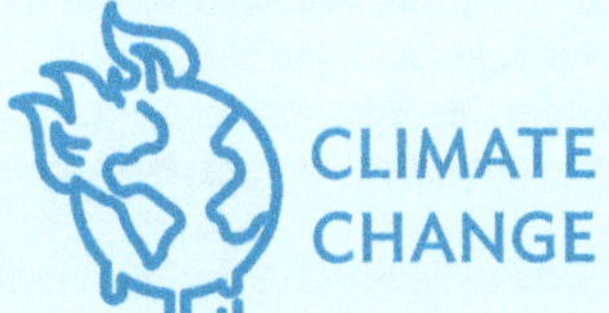

PREVENTION and **REDUCTION** of climate change

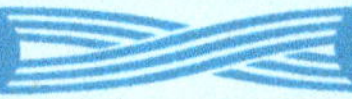

Source: Nossal Institute for Global Health, authors.

BOX 3

The Role of One Health in Global and Regional Climate Commitments

In 2015, 196 states agreed to reduce greenhouse gas emissions under the 2015 United Nations Framework Convention on Climate Change Paris Agreement.[a] As well as reining-in the effects of climate change, these reductions could yield significant health benefits.[b] Climate change mitigation policies, involving multiple sectors such as energy, construction, transport, and food and agriculture could bring about cleaner air, improved housing, increased physical activity, and healthier diets.[c]

The Asian Development Bank plays a key role in working with its developing member countries to meet their obligations under the Paris Agreement, and has declared itself to be the region's climate bank, committed to delivering $80 billion in cumulative climate financing from its own resources by 2030 and for at least 75% of its operations by number of projects to feature climate adaptation and mitigation initiatives.[d]

To meet its climate finance objectives, more projects will need to focus on activities that directly reduce physical climate risk. They will need to build the adaptive capacity of the system within which the activity takes place, addressing climate vulnerability at the project planning phase.

Using a One Health framework can support that integrated process. The One Health framework can help generate actions, and investments sectors such as water, agriculture, transport, energy, and health can work together toward shared goals, especially those relating to climate change.

The G20 has committed to strengthening global health and implementing a One Health approach, notably to tackle antimicrobial resistance, in collaboration with multilateral development banks to enhance the resilience of health systems and support development of climate resilient and low-carbon health.[e] Further, the G20 Climate and Health Initiative which was formally launched at COP 28 in late 2023, includes One Health in its key principles.

Sources:
[a] United Nations Climate Change. The Paris Agreement. What is the Paris Agreement?
[b] Gao J., Kovats S., Vardoulakis S., et al. 2018. Public health co-benefits of greenhouse gas emissions reduction: a systematic review. *Sci Total Environ.* 627. pp. 388–402.
[c] Hamilton I, et al. 2021. The Public Health Implications of the Paris Agreement: A Modelling Study. *The Lancet Planetary Health.* 5 (2). pp. E74–E83.
[d] ADB. 2021. ADB President Calls for "Bold Action" on Climate Change at 16th Asia Clean Energy Forum. Press Release. 15 June.
[e] Group of Twenty. G20 New Delhi Leaders' Declaration.

Threats to Biodiversity and Wildlife

When human use of land encroaches on wildlife habitats, it brings more species into contact with people, increasing the risk of zoonotic spillover. Reduced biodiversity, including through wildlife hunting and trade, also drives transmission of zoonotic diseases to humans.[19] Wildlife species become more vulnerable to viral diseases as they struggle to meet their need for food and shelter.[20]

---

[19] World Health Organization Regional Office for Europe. 2022. *A Health Perspective on the Role of the Environment in One Health.* Copenhagen.
[20] Kütükçü, A. E., Davas, A. Çağlayan, C., Tolunay, D., Gacal, F., Yavuz, M. 2021. *A One Health Approach to Climate Change and the COVID-19 Pandemic.* Health and Environment and Climate Turkey.

GMS countries share common wildlife issues, including relatively unregulated wildlife markets, known hotpots for zoonotic disease spread,[21] and illicit transboundary trade in wildlife.[22] Transboundary animal diseases pose serious threats to livelihoods, food security, trade, and economic growth.[23] In the GMS, they hamper productivity, cause market disruptions, and limit formal trade and market access to livestock suppliers, and as such are a key nontariff barrier to trade in live animals. By bringing together different stakeholders in human health, animal health, and trade, the One Health framework offers a way to resolve the risks associated with illegal wildlife trading, which takes into account the interests, strengths, and constraints of all three groups.

Antimicrobial Resistance

AMR is predicted to lead to over 47 million excess deaths in Asia by 2050, undermining progress in fighting infectious diseases and increasing health care costs.[24] Climate change is likely contributing to observed increases in AMR, by altering environmental conditions which may stimulate bacterial growth and horizontal gene transfer (the exchange of genetic material that can cause AMR), and accelerate the rate of resistance.[25] These AMR pathogens and genetic elements can pass between humans, animals, and the environment.

AMR affects both humans and livestock[26] and is a serious issue in the GMS.[27] This is not just in the case of artemisinin-resistant malaria,[28] but also antibiotic resistance due to misuse and irrational use in the animal and human health sectors.[29] Studies in the GMS have shown livestock, particularly poultry and pigs, are reared in farming systems that overly rely on use of antimicrobials for both growth promotion and treatment of diseases, contributing to increased occurrence of AMR.[30] GMS governments recognize the critical threat these hazards pose, as evidenced by the proliferation of food safety laws and AMR national action plans in the GMS (footnote 29). However, best practice antimicrobial use in livestock and effective regulation of antimicrobial importation and distribution are lacking.

Containing AMR is recognized as a global public health priority.[31] Even if the economic impact of AMR could only be halved through vigorous AMR containment efforts, the expected cumulative global benefits in 2017–2050 range between $10 trillion and $27 trillion, vs. investment costs of just $0.2 trillion, according to the World Bank.[32] Tackling AMR is an example of how a One Health framework can address a health issue affecting human, environmental, and animal health (Figure 4).[33]

[21] Aguirre A.A., Catherina R., Frye H., Shelley L. 2020. Illicit Wildlife Trade, Wet Markets, and COVID-19: Preventing Future Pandemics. *World Med Health Policy*. 3. pp. 256–265.

[22] Luong H.T., and Thomson N. 2022. *Trafficking in Contagion: Environmental Crime and Biological Threats in the Greater Mekong*. Global Initiative Against Transnational Crime.

[23] Clemmons, E.A.; Alfson, K.J.; Dutton, J.W., III. 2021. Transboundary Animal Diseases, an Overview of 17 Diseases with Potential for Global Spread and Serious Consequences. *Animals*. 11(17). p. 2039

[24] *Antimicrobial Resistance: Tackling a Crisis for the Health and Wealth of Nations*. 2014.

[25] Lio, R. M. S., et al. 2023. How Antimicrobial Resistance Is Linked to Climate Change: An Overview of Two Intertwined Global Challenges. *Int. J. Environ. Res. Public. Health*. 20. p. 1681.

[26] Murray, C. J. L., et al. 2022. Global Burden of Bacterial Antimicrobial Resistance in 2019: A Systematic Analysis. *The Lancet*. 399(10325). p. 629–655.

[27] Magnusson U., Moodley A., Osbjer K. 2021. Antimicrobial resistance at the livestock–human interface: implications for Veterinary Services. *Scientific & Technical Review*. 40(2). pp. 511–521.

[28] Asian Development Bank. ADB Regional Malaria and Other Communicable Disease Threats Trust Fund.

[29] Asian Development Bank and Nossal Institute for Global Health. *Operationalising One Health to Manage Antimicrobial Resistance and Support the Green Recovery*.

[30] Nhung, N., Cuong, N., Thwaites, G., and Carrique-Mas, J. 2016. Antimicrobial Usage and Antimicrobial Resistance in Animal Production in Southeast Asia: A Review. *Antibiotics-Basel*. 5.

[31] World Health Organization Antimicrobial Resistance. 2023. Key Facts. 21 November.

[32] Jonas, O. B., Irwin, Alec, Berthe, F. C. J., Le Gall, F. G. Marquez, P. V. 2017. Drug-Resistant Infections: A Threat to Our Economic Future (Vol. 2). Final Report (English). HNP/Agriculture Global Antimicrobial Resistance Initiative Washington, DC: World Bank Group.

[33] Velazquez-Meza ME, Galarde-López M, Carrillo-Quiróz B, Alpuche-Aranda CM. Antimicrobial resistance: One Health approach. Vet World. 2022 Mar;15(3):743-749. doi: 10.14202/vetworld.2022.743-749. Epub 2022 Mar 28.

Antimicrobial Resistance and One Health

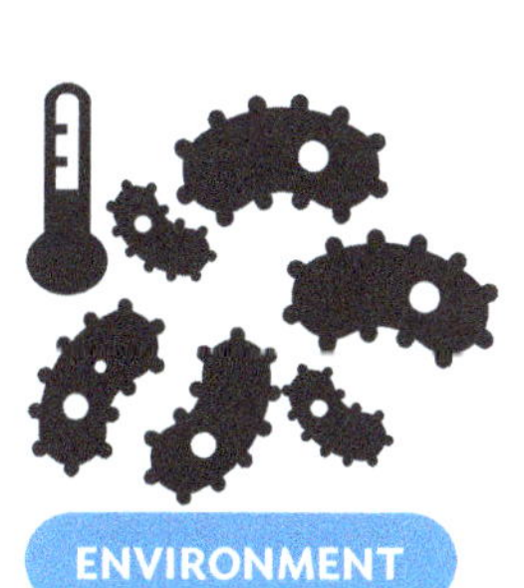

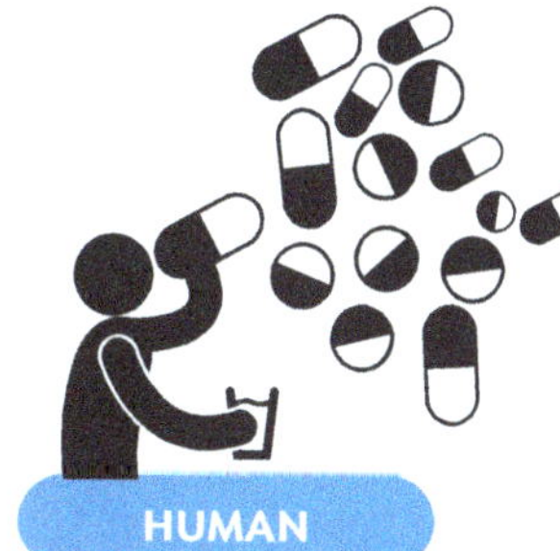

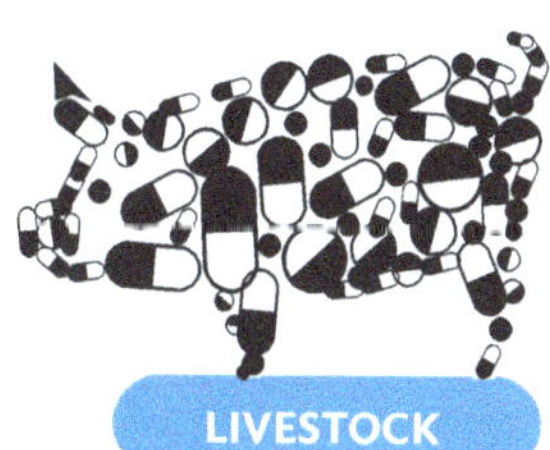

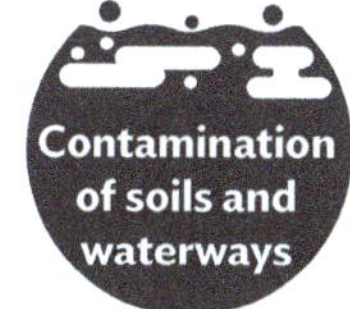

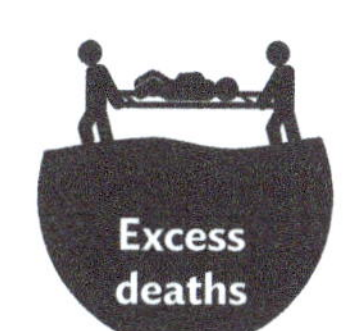

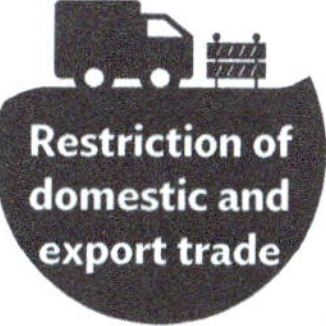

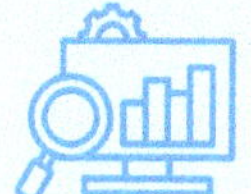

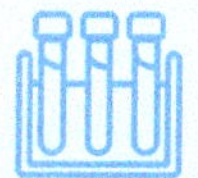

AMR = Antimicrobial resistance.
Source: Authors

Zoonotic Diseases

Climate change is altering the distribution, transmission, and severity of zoonotic pathogens.[34] It influences the geography of diseases, causing shifts in natural ecosystems that affect animal species' geographical range, vectors, reservoirs, and susceptible hosts.[35] Extreme weather events cause the movement of animals closer to human communities as they become displaced from their existing habitats, and can create conditions conducive to unusual clusters of zoonotic diseases.

Climate change may also be changing the geographic distribution of diseases such as Nipah virus.[36] Nipah virus outbreaks can have a huge economic toll. The 1998–1999 Nipah outbreak in Malaysia, for example, caused 265 cases of acute encephalitis leading to 105 deaths.[37] The outbreak led to the culling of over 1 million pigs, causing the near-collapse of the billion-dollar pig-farming industry.[38] An outbreak in Kerala, India in 2023 led to a public health lockdown. It was the first such lockdown in the case of a Nipah virus outbreak.[39] Natural disasters can lead to the spread of diseases, such as the reemergence of leptospirosis in the People's Republic of China (PRC) following Typhoon Nali in 2001.[40]

The GMS is home to a significant number of endemic zoonoses (Table 1) from bacterial diseases, such as anthrax and salmonellosis, to viral diseases such as avian influenza and rabies. These threaten entire communities, especially specific at-risk groups such as agriculture workers, pregnant women, and people who are immuno-compromised. Southeast Asian countries have high incidence of rabies due to the high number of unvaccinated stray and pet dogs, and in some settings (e.g., dog butchers in Viet Nam) due to work hazards. The low availability of rabies vaccines in rural areas and misinformation about importance of seeking timely treatment after dog bites are also contributory factors.[41] Rabies control is a classic example of the effectiveness of using a One Health framework (Box 4).[42]

On a larger scale, prevention is always better than cure. The World Bank estimates that switching from a reactive pandemic response to a proactive pandemic prevention strategy would cost between $10.3 billion and $11.5 billion a year with components for biosecurity, veterinary services, and deforestation reduction.[43] The World Bank estimates that these prevention costs are less than 1% of the cost of responding to COVID-19 pandemic in 2020.

Food Security and Safety

Food security and fresh water supplies are threatened by rising sea levels and increasing ocean temperatures, as well as heat waves and longer, more intense droughts.[44] Globally, there are growing concerns about long-term sustainability of food production.[45] More extreme weather events, such as floods and droughts caused by climate

[34]   Wolmuth-G. H., and Mutebi N. 2023. *Public Health and Climate Change: A One Health Approach.* The Parliamentary Office of Science and Technology. UK Houses of Parliament.

[35]   Berthe,F. C. J., Bali, S., R., Batmanian, G. J. 2022. *Putting Pandemics Behind Us: Investing in One Health to Reduce Risks of Emerging Infectious Diseases* (English). Washington, DC: World Bank Group.

[36]   Martin G., Yanez-Arenas C., Chen C., et al. 2018. Climate Change Could Increase the Geographic Extent of Hendra Virus Spillover Risk. *Ecohealth.*15. 509–25.

[37]   Looi L.M., Chua K.B. 2007. Lessons from the Nipah Virus Outbreak in Malaysia. *Malays J Pathol.* 29(2). pp. 63–7. PMID: 19108397.

[38]   Hosono, H., Kono, H., Ito, S., Shirai, J. 2006. Economic Impact of Nipah Virus Infection Outbreak in Malaysia. Obihiro University of Agriculture and Veterinary Medicine. National Institute of Animal Health Proceedings of the 11th International Symposium on Veterinary Epidemiology and Economics. Cairns Australia.

[39]   Johnson, T., Jamrozik, E., Hurst, T., et al. 2023. Ethical Issues in Nipah Virus Control and Research: Addressing a Neglected Disease. *Journal of Medical Ethics* Published Online 9 December.

[40]   Watson, J.T., Gayer, M., Connolly, M.A. 2007. Epidemics After Natural Disasters. *Emerg Infect Dis.* 13(1). pp. 1–5.

[41]   Ling, M. Y. J., Halim, A. F. N. A., Ahmad, D., et al. 2023. Rabies in Southeast Asia: A Systematic Review of its Incidence, Risk Factors and Mortality. *BMJ Open.* 13(5):e066587.

[42]   World Health Organization. 2013. WHO Expert Consultation on Rabies. Second report. *World Health Organ Tech Rep Ser.* 982. pp. 1–139.

[43]   World Bank. 2022. *Putting Pandemics Behind Us: Investing in One Health to Reduce Risks of Emerging Infectious Diseases.* Washington, DC: World Bank.

[44]   WWF. Effects of Climate Change.

[45]   United States Agency for International Development. 2022. USAID One Health Landscape Assessment. 12 October.

TABLE 1 Examples of Endemic Zoonoses in the Greater Mekong Subregion

Disease	Human Risk Groups	Animal Reservoir
Anthrax	Rural livestock-raising communities, animal health workers	Herbivores
Bovine (zoonotic) tuberculosis	Immuno-compromised, consumers of infected milk	Cattle, wild animals
Brucellosis	Pregnant women, farmers	Cattle, goats, sheep, pigs, dogs
Leptospirosis	Rice field workers, livestock workers	Wild and domestic animals including rodents, cattle
Salmonellosis	Young, old, pregnant, immune-compromised	Multiple species, especially food-producing animals
Streptococcus suis meningitis	Meat consumers, pig farmers, meat workers, immuno-compromised,	Multiple mammalian species, especially pigs
Avian influenza	Rural poultry producers & traders, women, children	Poultry, migratory waterfowl
Japanese encephalitis	Rural rice and pig farmers	Pigs, wild birds
Nipah virus disease	Bat hunters and consumers, farmers, health care workers	Fruit bats
Rabies	Children, rural poor, dog eaters	Domestic and wild carnivores, other mammals
Trichinosis	Rural adults and children, meat consumers	Pigs, rodents, dogs, cats, horses

Notes:
1. Sources of human infection: animal excreta; carcasses of infected animals; close physical contact with infected animals; contact with aborted fetuses, fetal membranes, and birth fluids; contaminated meat; food and water contaminated with the urine from infected animals; insects; milk.
2. Routes of human infection: contact with animals and animal products, contact with skin or mucosa, ingestion, inhalation, inoculation.

Source: Nossal Institute for Global Health.

BOX 4

Rabies Control Using a One Health Framework

The Indian state of Tamil Nadu pioneered a One Health Committee to address the challenge of rabies in dogs and humans and introduced a state-wide, multisectoral rabies control program. It comprised public health surveillance and awareness campaigns, animal census and implementation of dog licensing rules, waste management, combined dog sterilization and anti-rabies vaccination, and widespread availability of anti-rabies vaccine at all public health facilities.[a] In Tamil Nadu, controlling rabies infections in humans through dog vaccination was found to be not only highly feasible, but also cost-effective.[b]

[a] Abbas, S.S., Venkataramanan, V., Pathak, G., Kakkar, M. 2011. Roadmap to Combat Zoonoses in India (RCZI) Initiative. Rabies Control Initiative in Tamil Nadu, India: A Test Case for the 'One Health' Approach. *Int Health*. 3(4). pp. 231–9.
[b] H. Byrnes, Britton, A., Bhutia, T. 2017. Eliminating Dog-Mediated Rabies in Sikkim, India: A 10-Year Pathway to Success for the SARAH Program. *Front Vet Sci*. 4(28).
Source: Authors.

change are increasing the incidence of ruined crops, culled livestock, and livestock and crop disease.[46] Climate change can also affect water sanitation and hygiene, such as through contamination of water sources due to flooding. Higher temperatures also lead to increased incidence of foodborne infections.[47]

Livestock production is not only a source of high-quality nutritious food, but it also has economic benefits, provides employment, and contributes to economic development and trade.[48] In the GMS, food systems often lack the necessary infrastructure for effective disease monitoring and control, and value chains in the subregion are complex, fragmented, relatively inefficient and frequently cross borders. Poor facilities for slaughtering, cold storage, and processing contribute to poor food safety, high food wastage, and low competitiveness (footnote 29). By investing in infrastructure such as animal disease control zones, effective veterinary services, diagnostic laboratories, and quarantine facilities, it is possible to improve livelihoods, resilience, and food security in the GMS, and at the same time reduce public health risks.

Applying One Health approaches to food systems would provide entry points to address many of the emerging and global public health threats in the GMS (Figure 5). Examples include taking into account animal diseases and the risk for transmission of zoonotic pathogens when conducting food value chain risk assessments; implementing quality assurance programs to both reduce foodborne disease risks and support improved productivity and safety for the livestock sector; and implementing programs that reduce the risk of animal-to-human disease transmission through markets and other livestock aggregation points such as collection yards, live animal markets, and slaughterhouses.

---

[46] Intergovernmental Panel on Climate Change. Core Writing Team; Lee, H. and Romero, J., eds. 2023. *Climate Change 2023: Synthesis Report. Contribution of Working Groups I, II and III to the Sixth Assessment Report of the Intergovernmental Panel on Climate Change.* IPCC: Geneva, Switzerland. pp. 35–115.

[47] World Health Organization Regional Office for Europe. 2022. *A Health Perspective on the Role of the Environment in One Health.* Copenhagen.

[48] Srinivasan, A. 2023. Building Resilience in the Greater Mekong Subregion's Agri-Food Sector. *Development Asia.* Manila: Asian Development Bank.

FIGURE 5

One Health Approaches to Food Safety and Security

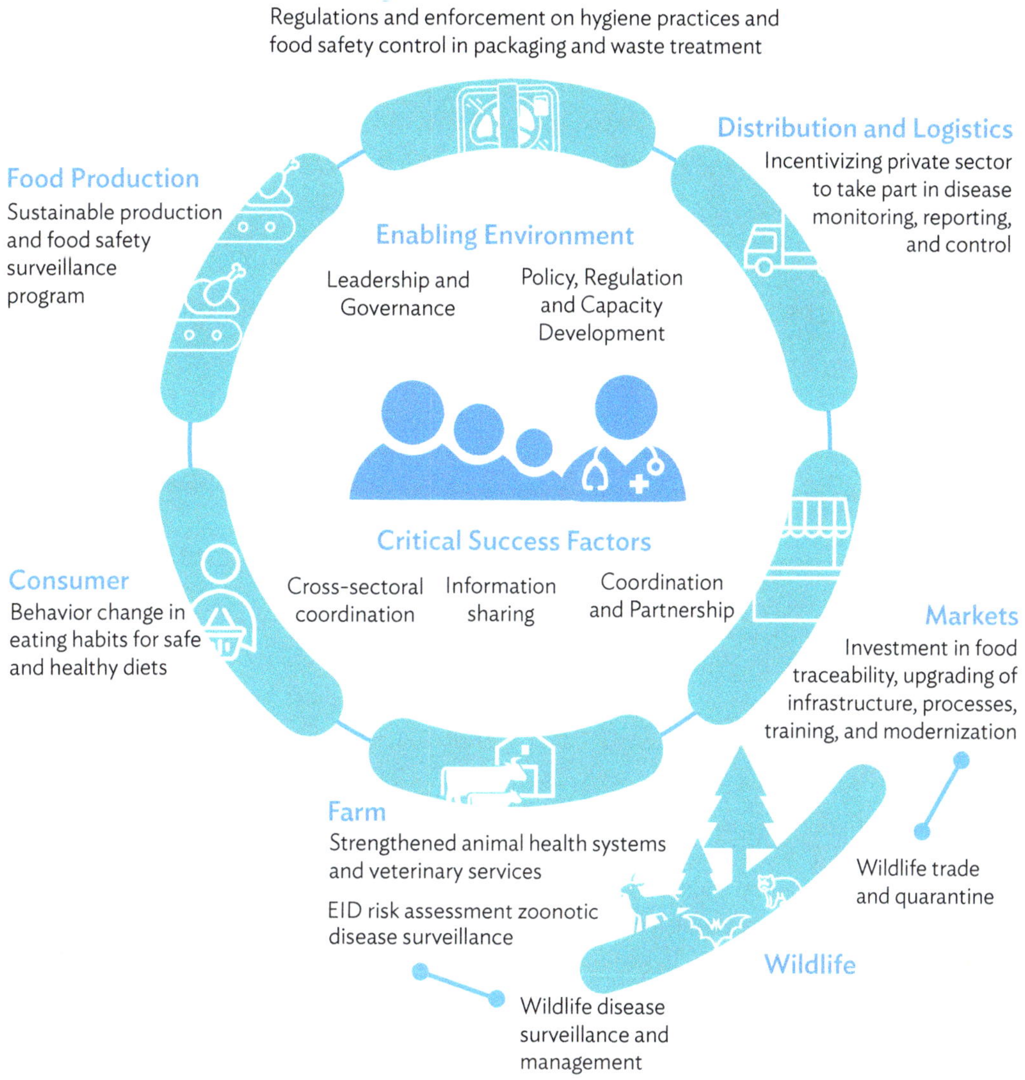

Source: World Bank and Food and Agriculture Organization (FAO). 2022. *From Reacting to Preventing Pandemics - Building Animal Health and Wildlife Systems for One Health in East Asia and Pacific*. Washington, DC: World Bank and FAO.

2 ONE HEALTH ACTIVITIES IN THE GREATER MEKONG SUBREGION

Support for the Greater Mekong Subregion

GMS countries have already made explicit commitments to adopting a One Health approach. *The Greater Mekong Subregion Economic Cooperation Program Strategic Framework 2030* (GMS-2030) positions health security as a regional public good.[49] It calls for a unified view of animal and human diseases and their interactions, and for upgrading cross-border cooperation instruments and intraregional and multisectoral collaboration. One Health is one of the ways in which this can be operationalized, including through ASEAN One Health initiatives (see Box 1, p. 4).

GMS-2030 states: "action will focus on developing governance frameworks for the operational linking of health and non-health sectors, building animal health system capacity to align with that of public health systems, and harmonizing food safety systems. Opportunities to build on existing One Health programs, including those linking veterinary and public health workforce and veterinary and human health laboratory networks will be explored." GMS-2030 provides the setting for the development of the subregion for the next decade. It recommends a unified approach to environmental, animal, and human health under One Health, and the need for strengthening the performance of GMS health systems to prevent, detect, and respond to public health threats and emerging diseases.

Understanding the Current State of One Health in the Greater Mekong Subregion

In response to the impact of COVID-19 pandemic, ADB expanded the regional technical assistance (TA) 9571 Supporting Health Cooperation in the Greater Mekong Subregion in February 2020 to include "Scaling Up One Health Approaches in the GMS." Under this TA, ADB commissioned the Nossal Institute for Global Health at the University of Melbourne to promote One Health principles to strengthen health security in the GMS. The Nossal Institute's work, undertaken from July 2020 to January 2023, included

---

[49]   Asian Development Bank. 2021. *Greater Mekong Subregion Economic Cooperation Program Strategic Framework 2030*. Manila.

- a comprehensive assessment of the current state of One Health principles in the GMS;
- development of a strategic framework for implementing One Health principles in the region;
- exploring potential collaborations between academic institutions and international organizations to promote health security and strengthen One Health initiatives;
- development of a case to support One Health investments; and
- a knowledge platform for sharing and capacity building on One Health principles among health care professionals and policymakers.

The Nossal Institute research revealed high awareness of the concept of One Health in the GMS. This can be partly attributed to that 2003 SARS epidemic, and ongoing outbreaks of highly pathogenic avian influenzas, which have occurred in the GMS since the early 2000s, and more recently the COVID-19 pandemic.[50] Although One Health initiatives are at different stages of evolution across all six countries (see country profiles) and each has their own specific challenges, they also share some common features such as the threat of transboundary animal diseases. The regional mapping undertaken by Nossal Institute showcased several organizations and initiatives aimed at strengthening the region's capacity to respond to health emergencies using a One Health approach. However, poor coordination and collaboration among partners, combined with inadequate resources, has undermined the impact of past One Health initiatives. Future regional TA has great potential to support regional initiatives driven by academia, civil society, technical bodies, and possibly the private sector.

Outside the government sector, there is strong interest in One Health from academia, with One Health university networks active in all four countries and with connection to other colleagues through the Southeast Asia Regional One Health University Network.[51] Engagement with nongovernment organizations (NGOs) and civil society varies from country to country, and the private sector is an under-engaged source of partnership and collaboration. The Southeast Asia One Health University Network (SEAOHUN), established in 2011 with support from the One Health Workforce project of the United States Agency for International Development (USAID), One Health Workforce project, has members from across the GMS. This network could play a role under a future TA and their active involvement on regional One Health activities should be encouraged.

Regional One Health Implementation: Activities, Gaps, Opportunities

The GMS Working Group on One Health is co-led by the ministers of health for Cambodia, the Lao People's Democratic Republic (Lao PDR), Myanmar, the PRC, Thailand, and Viet Nam, and has committed to advance implementation of One Health actions.[52] This commitment was confirmed through several seminars held during the COVID-19 pandemic, with participation from a broad range of stakeholders representing different sectors, including environment, agriculture, and human health. The new GMS Health Cooperation Strategy 2024–2030 will also reconfirm the importance of scaling up One Health actions in the region. Separately, the GMS working groups on environment and agriculture have also expressed interest in joint work on One Health in the GMS.

All six countries of the GMS either have a national One Health strategy or are in the process of developing one (Table 2). The most common collaboration so far has been between human and animal health at central and local level, typically around zoonotic disease control and surveillance. National awareness is high but maintaining momentum at subnational and local levels has proven to be difficult. Collaboration between the environmental sector and the human–animal health sectors is underdeveloped across the region. Similarly, responsibility for wildlife issues is often fragmented among several ministries with heavy reliance on donor-led projects—often making it difficult for getting the sector comprehensively engaged with One Health projects.

---

[50] World Health Organization Regional Office for Europe. 2023. *How Coronavirus Disease has Changed the Environment and Health Landscape.* Web Annex: A Rapid Review of Reviews. Copenhagen.
[51] Southeast Asia Regional One Health University Network.
[52] ADB has placed a temporary hold on sovereign project disbursements and new contracts in Myanmar effective 1 February 2021.

TABLE 2 **National Action and Strategic Plans**

	One Health	Antimicrobial Resistance
Cambodia	One Health Joint Plan of Action 2022[a]	Multi-Sectoral Action Plan on Antimicrobial Resistance 2019–2023.[b]
People's Republic of China	No[g]	China: Second national action plan for containing antimicrobial resistance 2022-2025.[h]
Lao PDR	No[c]	Lao PDR: National strategic plan on antimicrobial resistance in Lao PDR 2019-2023.[d]
Myanmar	No[e]	Myanmar National Action Plan for Containment of Antimicrobial Resistance (2017-2022).[f]
Thailand	Thailand National strategic Plan for Emerging Infectious Disease (2017-2021)[i] adopted One Health approach[j]	Thailand's National Strategic Plan on Antimicrobial Resistance 2017-2021.[k]
Viet Nam	Master Plan for the One Health Partnership Framework for Zoonoses, 2021 – 2025 Period[l]	National Action Plan on Combatting Drug Resistance 2013–2020[m]
		National Action Plan for management of antibiotic use and control of antibiotic resistance in livestock production and aquaculture 2017-2020[n]

[a] *Khmer Times*. 2022. One Health Joint Plan of Action launched to address health threats to humans, animals, plants and environment. 18 October.
[b] Food and Agriculture Organization of the United Nations. 2019. *Cambodia: Multi-Sectoral Action Plan on Antimicrobial Resistance 2019-2023*.
[c] National Bridging Workshop for One Health – Lao PDR. 2023. Vang Vieng, Lao People's Democratic Republic. 9–11 August.
[d] World Health Organization. 2019. *Lao PDR: National Strategic Plan on Antimicrobial Resistance in Lao PDR 2019–2023*.
[e] One Health MYANMAR.
[f] Food and Agriculture Organization of the United Nations. 2017. *Myanmar National Action Plan for Containment of Antimicrobial Resistance (2017–2022)*.
[g] Jing-Shu Liu, Xin-Chen Li, Qi-Yu Zhang, Le-Fei Han, et al. 2023. China's application of the One Health approach in addressing public health threats at the human-animal-environment interface: Advances and challenges. *One Health*. 17. 100607.
[h] World Health Organization. 2022. *China: Second national action plan for containing antimicrobial resistance 2022-2025*.
[i] Tangwangvivat, R. One Health in Thailand.
[j] Sommanustweechai A, Iamsirithaworn S, Patcharanarumol, et al. 2017. Adoption of One Health in Thailand's National Strategic Plan for Emerging Infectious Diseases. *J Public Health Policy*. 38(1). pp. 121–136.
[k] Food and Agriculture Organization of the United Nations. 2017. *Thailand's National Strategic Plan on Antimicrobial Resistance 2017-2021*.
[l] Government of Viet Nam, Ministry of Health. 2022. Master Plan for the One Health Partnership Framework for Zoonoses, 2021–2025 Period. Ha Noi.
[m] World Health Organization. 2013. *Vietnam: National action plan for combating drug resistance*.
[n] Government of Viet Nam, Ministry of Agriculture and Rural Development. 2017. *National Action Plan for Management of Antibiotic Use and Control of Antibiotic Resistance in Livestock Production and Aquaculture*. Ha Noi.

Source: Compiled by authors.

National One Health Implementation: Activities, Gaps, Opportunities

Cambodia

At country level, it is the Cambodian working group on health that is the most active, with its work fully funded by the United Nations (UN) Quadripartite and development partners, leading to the development of a comprehensive work plan for One Health. German state-owned investment and development bank KfW, in partnership with WHO and the Ministry of Health in Cambodia, has initiated the One Health 4 Cambodia project. This initiative aims to create an overarching One Health architecture focusing on three areas: reduction of AMR, risk reduction for disease spillover from wildlife and animal husbandry, and the infectious disease and/or climate interface, including how taking climate into consideration can improve pandemic, emerging infection disease and AMR forecasting, modeling and response.

There is an existing mechanism for communicable disease surveillance, the Cambodia Early Warning Alert and Response Network, a multi-source, case-based surveillance system for seven common disease symptoms. This system can detect zoonotic infections, but it creates a lot of noise that may weaken these signals, as its symptom-based reporting requirements also pick up clusters of food, pesticide, and alcohol poisoning. However, the system is in place to detect outbreaks of zoonotic disease, and could be improved, through more funding for rapid field investigations, for example.

The Cambodia Zoonoses Technical Working group brings together stakeholders from the Ministry of Agriculture, Forestry and Fisheries and the Ministry of Health during outbreaks of zoonotic disease, but it is also hampered by inadequate funding. It is currently inactive, and there is no automated mechanism for data sharing.

Acute workforce shortages affect Cambodia's ability to develop a One Health-competent workforce, with the government veterinary workforce, for example, in decline as young people eschew such careers for urban employment. The private sector remains an untapped source of capacity for One Health in Cambodia, together with civil society. The recently formed Cambodia One Health University Network, comprising five Cambodian universities, has a 2020–2025 strategic plan and a mission to develop a sustainable network of One Health professionals with cross-sectoral expertise.

Lao People's Democratic Republic

The Lao PDR is in the process of creating a national One Health Committee, which will build on previous efforts to coordinate activities. The country has national preparedness and response plans for numerous human diseases, and a Joint Contingency Plan for avian influenza, but actual outbreak investigations and response are infrequent, and capacity is limited. In the human health sector, the system is hampered by using a combination of paper-based and digital reporting.

In the animal sector, there is no surveillance system for some priority zoonotic diseases, and communication with the health sector about outbreaks of zoonotic disease relies on informal relationships. Laboratory capacity for human health has undergone improvements, but these have not been matched in the animal health sector. Currently only two of five national priority zoonoses (highly pathogenic avian influenza and rabies) are actively investigated and there is much scope for improvement of the surveillance and reporting system. Beyond disease response, efforts to operationalize One Health are at the mercy of the priorities of discrete externally funding projects such as the USAID- and FAO-supported Global Health Security Agenda and the Lao PDR-Cambodia One Health Surveillance and Laboratory Network. The Lao One Health University Network, covering five Lao PDR universities, supports strategic capacity building for One Health.

The Lao PDR is increasingly connected to regional animal trading networks, and to their associated efforts to reduce the risk of transboundary animal diseases. The country has previously participated in cross-border zoonotic disease surveillance with Thailand, but this suffered from a lack of investment from the Lao PDR side. Investment support for regional participation would strengthen cross-border disease control and sector development.

Regionally, the Lao PDR is one of the most biodiverse countries in Southeast Asia, but this has been negatively impacted by deforestation and trade of economically valuable wildlife from its forests to markets in the PRC and Viet Nam, a recognized driver of infectious disease emergence. strengthening One Health joint activities in biodiversity and protected areas management and regulating (or preventing) wildlife trade is important for addressing emerging infectious disease threats for the wider GMS.

Thailand

One Health Capacity
With more than 2 decades' experience in implementing One Health activities, Thailand is at the forefront of this work in the GMS. From the top down, Thailand has embedded a One Health approach in national legislation, strategic plans, and policies at multiple levels of government, and in partnership with NGOs and civil society. It has invested in One Health leadership courses for mid-level government staff. One Health was the designated basis for implementation of the 2013–2016 National Strategic Plan for Emerging Infectious Diseases: Preparedness, Prevention and Response.

In 2014, the National Committee on Emerging Infectious Disease Preparedness and Response established the Coordinating Unit for One Health, housed in the Ministry of Public Health, but operating autonomously, and steered by a committee drawn from human, animal, wildlife, and environmental ministries, as well as academia and international organizations. The 2017–2021 National Strategic Plan for Emerging Infectious Diseases was also grounded in One Health principles. There are at least 22 institutions actively engaged in One Health in Thailand. The Thailand One Health University Network has a particularly extensive national membership comprising medical and veterinary faculties and universities throughout the country.

One Health Operationalization
Thailand has protocols for both national and international data sharing on routine surveillance and public health emergencies and there are five priority diseases for this: rabies, zoonotic avian influenza, coronaviruses, Ebola virus disease, and Nipah virus disease. Thailand is the only GMS country that conducts integrated One Health surveillance for Nipah virus, an emerging infectious disease that has never been detected in humans in Thailand.

Although Thailand is well ahead of other GMS countries in One Health operationalization, it is still heavily focused on human health, and many programs only initiate disease control once a human case has been detected. Thailand's 1 million community-based health volunteers have been integral to surveillance and response efforts for decades and played a crucial role in the COVID-19 pandemic response. Similarly, the village livestock volunteer program of the Department of Livestock Development manages animal health workers in approximately 30,000 villages who support surveillance and outbreak response efforts, in addition to routine health and production issues. However, limited resources hamper the operationalization of One Health activities at provincial and district levels in Thailand, undermining their long-term sustainability.

Regional Linkages
Thailand plays an important role in strengthening One Health capacity in the GMS. It hosts regional One Health workforce development, promotes regional data-sharing initiatives, and supports capacity development for the prevention and control of transboundary and emerging infectious diseases in neighboring countries. Given that Thailand is a major destination for formal and informal migration in the GMS, and there is significant movement of livestock across Thailand's land borders, Thailand's role as an active regional implementer of One Health is especially important.

Thailand's regional contributions includes hosting the Regional Field Epidemiology Training Program for Veterinarians, an innovative and long-standing program established in close collaboration with the Ministry of Public Health that provides training for veterinarians from Thailand and 11 other countries, including all GMS countries. Thailand also hosts the regional base for the implementing agency of the Fleming Fund Regional Grants to address AMR throughout the region, and hosts the Monitoring and Surveillance Centre for Zoonotic Diseases in Wildlife and Exotic Animals, a national and regional reference center for zoonosis surveillance in wildlife.

Viet Nam

One Health Capacity

Viet Nam's second One Health Partnership Framework (OHP) for Zoonoses, 2021–2025, has 33 signatories within and outside government.[53] Since its inception, the OHP has been instrumental in the preparation and implementation of nearly 100 programs and projects. These include initiatives on collaborative wildlife disease surveillance, AMR, veterinary drug management, and active surveillance of bacteria in livestock.

The 2022 National Master Plan for the One Health Partnership Framework aims to operationalize the OHP framework, emphasizing the need for collaboration across agriculture, health, and the environment. The master plan targets the reduction of zoonotic diseases, environmental contributions to the risk of disease transmission to humans, and takes steps to combat AMR. This commitment materialized through six core areas of focus, reflecting a comprehensive strategy to safeguard public health.[54]

One Health Operationalization

The Ministry of Health has established a unified national steering committee to operationalize a One Health approach on a national scale. The Department of Animal Health runs the Viet Nam Animal Health Information System, which enables real-time reporting of suspected zoonotic disease cases and outbreaks in animals and the system now collects disease reports from all 63 provinces in Viet Nam.

Meanwhile, the health ministry collects data using the DHIS2 system. (a tool for collection, validation, analysis, and presentation of aggregate and patient-based statistical data). The human and animal data systems are not interoperable, and there are no established systems for routine sharing of relevant data. The government is exploring ways to address this, and there are also ongoing efforts to link wildlife and domestic animal disease surveillance and reporting.

Viet Nam has undertaken an external assessment of their veterinary services through the WOAH Performance of Veterinary Services Pathway and an assessment of compliance with the IHR 2005 through the WHO JEE Program. In 2023, the National Bridging Workshop was conducted to provide an opportunity for human health, animal health and environmental health services of the country to review their current collaboration gaps in key technical areas and to develop a joint road map of corrective measures and strategic investments to improve the collaborative work at the animal–human–environment interface.

An example of successful One Health surveillance in the livestock sector is Viet Nam's establishment of an integrated influenza surveillance network of humans, livestock, and wildlife in three high-risk provinces. Active surveillance for avian influenza now occurs at nearly 40% of live bird markets in Viet Nam, with H5N1, H5N6, and H9 subtypes frequently detected in poultry. As a result, in the past 5 years, small outbreaks among poultry were successfully controlled without extensive spread, and no human cases were recorded. To date, no H7N9 viruses have been detected in Viet Nam, unlike the situation in some neighboring countries.

Regional Linkages

Viet Nam also co-leads the Zoonotic Diseases Action Package of the Global Health Security Agenda, a 70-country consortium to strengthen global preparedness and response to infectious diseases with the potential to cause public health emergencies of national and international significance. Viet Nam's academic sector engages in One Health through the Vietnam One Health University Network (www.vohun.org) and participation in the SEAOHUN.

---

[53] Government of Viet Nam, Ministry of Agriculture and Rural Development. 2022. Master Plan for the One Health Partnership Framework for Zoonoses 2021–2025, Promulgated together with Decision No. 1039/QD-BNN-HTQT. 21 March 21.

[54] Government of Viet Nam, Ministry of Agriculture and Rural Development. 2023. No. /TT-HTQT-DP Report on the Results of the "Annual High-Level Forum 2023 of the One Health Partnership for Zoonoses 2021-2025 [Annual Report]." Ha Noi: Ministry of Agriculture and Rural Development. 15 November.

Cross-Sectoral Collaboration

Although every GMS country had a multisector information-sharing mechanisms, and most also have joint surveillance and response capacity, there are many gaps in resources (including infrastructure, human resources, and institutional capacity), as well as suboptimal engagement with the private sector, subnational levels of government, civil society, and communities.

Data sharing

There are complex legal nuances to data sharing that need to be considered, including whether the country has the necessary legislation in place for sharing of surveillance info between the animal and human health sectors. Moreover, it requires standardization and interoperability of information systems, with a standard set of metadata, to facilitate routine reporting. There needs to be a substantial enough laboratory information management system in the various sectors to facilitate sample information metadata and testing results, with sufficient interoperability, and a data access permission mechanism to determine what information is available to whom.

Coordination mechanisms

Thailand and Viet Nam are at the forefront of developing high-level, cross-sectoral One Health coordination mechanisms. Since 2003, Viet Nam has progressively embraced a multisectoral approach to tackle zoonotic diseases in response to domestic threats like highly pathogenic avian influenza and global initiatives promoting One Health. National planning has evolved from addressing avian influenza to a broader focus on emerging diseases and, finally, to a comprehensive national One Health road map—the Viet Nam OHP.

Legislation

Legislation has played a crucial role in fostering cooperation between animal and human health sectors, providing a legal framework for reporting notifiable infectious diseases, managing animal health, ensuring food safety, and responding to potential novel pathogens. Additionally, regulations have been introduced to manage captive wildlife, combat trafficking, and protect biodiversity. The key legal foundation for this cross-sectoral collaboration is provided by the Joint Circular (Circular No. 16/2013),[55] which facilitates coordination, information-sharing, and collaboration between the human and animal sectors in surveillance and response activities. However, despite awareness of these mechanisms, a recent survey revealed gaps in the practical application of One Health in the field and underscored a significant capacity gap (human resources, training, budget) as a key reason for problems with implementation of One Health.[56]

Veterinary, human and environmental health collaboration

Thailand has Coordinating Unit for One Health and Viet Nam has OHP. In Cambodia and the Lao PDR, this coordination is yet to be established. Potentially, international agencies, such as the Institut Pasteur can support One Health coordination mechanisms, by bridging activities across sectors and bringing capacity in disease diagnosis, surveillance, and research. In Cambodia, WHO is coordinating One Health work, convening One Health UN Quadripartite agencies, bilateral and multilateral development organizations, and other stakeholders to promote consensus on how to collaborate and better support the government on One Health areas. The focus is primarily on the area of human health, i.e., food safety, AMR, and zoonoses.

---

[55] Government of Viet Nam, Ministry of Health Ministry of Agriculture and Rural Development. 2013. The Joint Circular No. 16/2013/TTLT-BYT-BNN-PTNT Guiding Joint Activities for Prevention and Control of Animal Disease. 27 May.

[56] Auplish A., Vu, T.T.T., Pham Duc, P., Green, A., Tiwari, H., et al. 2024 Capacity and Needs Assessment of Veterinary Services in Vietnam in Biosecurity, Biosafety and One Health. *Plos One.* 19(1): e0295898.

Disease surveillance and reporting systems are largely absent from wildlife farming, despite the sector's rapid growth and critical importance in disease spillover risk.[57] NGOs such as the Wildlife Conservation Society, and international projects like the USAID PREDICT project have supported government surveillance in wild animals in Cambodia, the Lao PDR, and Viet Nam, but this work is not yet sustainably institutionalized or resourced.[58]

Across the region, the environmental sector is the least represented in One Health mechanisms and activities for a variety of reasons. In some countries, this is due to budget, staff, and other resource limitations. Environment sector operations, such as disease reporting, are often not integrated into those of the other sectors. In some countries, inclusion of environmental sector activities in One Health is complicated by different activities falling under the responsibility of different ministries, leading to fragmentation of efforts. For example, wildlife health might be included in One Health coordination because animal health is overseen by the Ministry of Agriculture but other One Health activities in the environment sector, such as environmental monitoring of pharmaceutical residues, are less coordinated across sectors.[59]

There are complex legal nuances to data sharing that need to be considered, including whether the country has the necessary legislation in place for sharing of surveillance info between the animal and human health sectors.

---

[57]   Nossal Institute. Current Status and Future Directions for One Health in the Greater Mekong Subregion.
[58]   United States Agency for International Development. Predict.
[59]   Campbell, A., Strachan, C., Barot B., et al. Scaling Up One Health Approaches in the Greater Mekong Subregion. Nossal Institute Final Report under RETA9571.

Foundations for Future One Health Work

GMS countries have existing infrastructure that could be built upon, such as joint surveillance networks, multisectoral cooperation strategies, or existing interministerial collaboration and data sharing (Table 3).

All six countries recognize that they have much to gain from regional cooperation and there is evidence of many efforts to do this, but it is challenging, because of the inherent tension between different countries' interests, despite their shared concerns.

Seen another way, the gaps in One Health across the GMS represent opportunities for quick wins in One Health strengthening, through improving existing networks and building human resource capacity, and improving communication with both communities and stakeholders. These opportunities are part of a broader business case for investments in One Health approaches.

TABLE 3 — Summary of One Health Mechanisms, Activities, and Focus on the Greater Mekong Subregion

Country	Cambodia	Lao PDR	Myanmar	PRC (Yunnan, Guangxi)	Thailand	Viet Nam
Mechanisms and Structures						
National One Health Committee or Working Group	✓	*	✓		✓	✓
Specific One Health National Unit or Plan	*		✓		✓	✓
Communicable Disease Control Department/Center						
Human CDC	✓	✓		✓	✓	
Animal CDC				✓	✓	
Combined CDC		✓			✓	
Ongoing funding				✓	✓	
Multisectoral Coordination						
Information-sharing	✓	✓	✓	✓	✓	✓
Joint surveillance	✓	✓		✓	✓	✓
Joint response	✓	✓		✓	✓	✓
Multisectoral Coordination: Focus Areas						
Zoonotic diseases	✓	✓	✓	✓	✓	✓
One Health	✓		✓	✓	✓	✓
Environmental management				✓	✓	
External Assessments						
Joint External Evaluation (WHO)	✓	✓	✓		✓	✓
Performance of Veterinary Services (WOAH)	✓	✓	✓		✓	✓
One Health National Bridging Workshop			✓		✓	

CDC = Centers for Disease Control, PRC = People's Republic of China, Lao PDR = Lao People's Democratic Republic, WHO = World Health Organization, WOAH = World Organisation for Animal Health.
* Under revision or development.

Source: Nossal Institute.

Summary of Key One Health Gaps Across the Greater Mekong Subregion

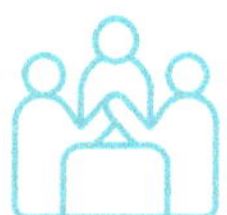

Limited One Health engagement with subnational levels of government (e.g., provincial, district), civil society, private sector, and communities

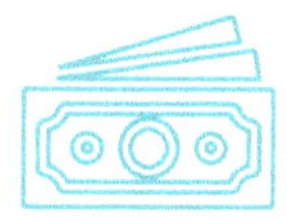

Dependence on external financing from donor-funded projects

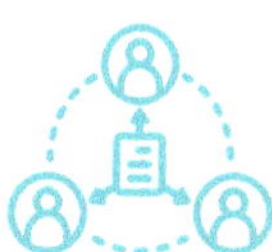

Siloed (non-interoperable) human and animal data systems and limited routine sharing of relevant data

Underdeveloped collaboration between the environmental sector and the human–animal health sectors

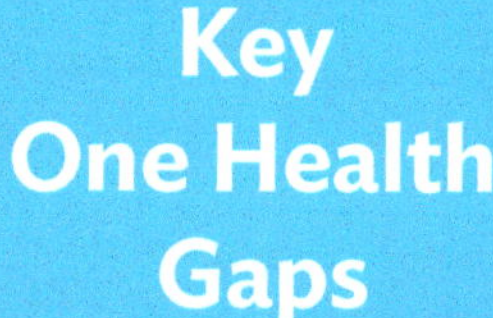

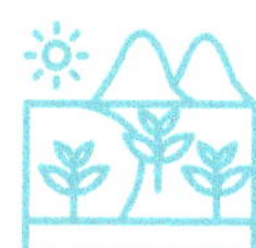

Fragmented responsibility for wildlife issues among several ministries

Limited One Health-competent workforce

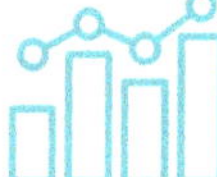

Limited capacity to conduct outbreak investigations and response

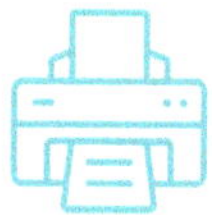

Parallel use of electronic and paper-based reporting

Source: Authors.

3 ONE HEALTH IN ADB OPERATIONS AND OPPORTUNITIES FOR ACTION

One Health aligns with the operational priorities of the ADB Strategy 2030—the bank's organizational strategy,[60] as well as its commitment to being a climate bank. Strategy 2030 focuses on achieving a prosperous, inclusive, resilient, and sustainable Asia and the Pacific. While not explicitly mentioned, key components of Strategy 2030 closely align with One Health principles, including poverty reduction, gender equality, climate change mitigation, disaster resilience, environmental sustainability, livable cities, rural development, and food security.

ADB is actively engaged in One Health activities, both implicitly and explicitly, through projects addressing human and animal health, antimicrobial usage and resistance, climate change, environment, and food safety and security across Asia and the Pacific. ADB's involvement is reflected in strategic documents guiding its actions and investments within regional subprograms.

- In the Central Asia Regional Cooperation Program Health Strategy 2030, One Health is listed as one of the guiding principles for the program and includes discussion of the need for surveillance for zoonoses and AMR, reporting of surveillance data through regional dashboards, and facilitating regional cross-border collaboration on zoonoses perhaps including establishment of a One Health regional institute.[61]
- Although the South Asia Subregional Economic Cooperation (SASEC) Operational Plan 2016–2025 does not explicitly mention health, climate, pandemic, and disaster resilience were all recently added to the program's list of operational priorities during the 2022 meeting of nodal officials.[62] Strengthening Regional Health Security through the One Health Approach is one of six new initiatives awaiting endorsement at the SASEC Finance Ministers Meeting.[63] This initiative aims to improve the coordination of SASEC country responses and minimize future disruptions to trade flows through regional disease surveillance and exchange of information.

[60] Asian Development Bank. 2018. *Strategy 2030: Achieving a Prosperous, Inclusive, Resilient, and Sustainable Asia and the Pacific.* Manila.
[61] Asian Development Bank. 2022. *CAREC Health Strategy 2030.*
[62] Asian Development Bank. South Asia Subregional Economic Cooperation (SASEC)
[63] SASEC. *Action Plan for SASEC Initiatives 2022–2024.*

In 2022, ADB published *Practical Actions to Operationalize the One Health Approach in the Asian Development Bank*, outlining how the organization can align with global One Health developments. This report provides a comprehensive framework for ADB to achieve its outcomes in harmony with One Health principles, emphasizing disaster risk mitigation, institution and governance enhancement, gender equality, and climate change mitigation, all crucial components of Strategy 2030. The One Health approach is seen as instrumental in achieving ADB's overarching targets, particularly in gender equality and climate change, reinforcing the principle of cross-sectoral collaboration within the organization.

ADB Projects with One Health Elements in the Greater Mekong Subregion

Under ADB's Greater Mekong Subregion Health Security Project, ADB has supported Cambodia, the Lao PDR, Myanmar, and Viet Nam with laboratory equipment and capacity building for One Health, including AMR under a regional loan project.[64] The loan project also supported operational costs for outbreak response and surveillance related to One Health and has supported regional meetings and workshops on disease surveillance and outbreak response related to One Health (e.g., influenza, food and mouth disease, and Nipah virus) under a regional TA project for all six GMS countries.[65]

There are other regional projects where ADB is already working at the human health–agriculture nexus, including the regional Greater Mekong Subregion Sustainable Agriculture and Food Security Program. Some of this project's outputs relate to human health, such as activities on food safety and quality standards; information exchange, coordination, and food risk communication strategies; and cross-border animal health and value chains capacity strengthening for animal health workers to control transboundary animal diseases and AMR.[66] ADB's Cambodia: Greater Mekong Subregion Cross-Border Livestock Health and Value Chains Improvement Project is a further example of ADB's growing use of One Health approaches to development (Box 5).

BOX 5

Realizing a Vision of Safe and Environmentally Friendly Agriculture in Cambodia

The Cambodia: Greater Mekong Subregion Cross-Border Livestock Health and Value Chains Improvement Project, comprising $93 million in loans and $12.9 million in grants, aims to reduce risks from transboundary animal diseases, build up animal health monitoring and service delivery, improve food safety, and promote subregional cooperation on climate-smart livestock production in the Greater Mekong Subregion.

While livestock production, health, trade, and food safety are all national strategic priorities in Cambodia, they have yet to be matched by adequate investments in livestock disease control infrastructure, capacity building, and enabling policies. The project will support adoption of a value chain approach, prioritizing integration of smallholders. The project will not only benefit Cambodia, but also its neighbors through regional cooperation and integration. It will promote private sector investments into livestock value chains through public–private partnerships by promoting conducive policies and supportive institutions.

By promoting trade and regional public goods, including regional health security, the project will also contribute to One Health objectives, and is a useful entry point to engage the government on this approach.

Source: ADB. 2022. Cambodia: Greater Mekong Subregion Cross-Border Livestock Health and Value Chains Improvement Project.

---

64   Asian Development Bank. Regional: Greater Mekong Subregion Health Security Project.
65   Asian Development Bank. Regional: Strengthening Regional Health Cooperation in the Greater Mekong Subregion.
66   Asian Development Bank. Regional: Greater Mekong Subregion Sustainable Agriculture and Food Security Program

The GMS Health Cooperation Strategy

The GMS Health Cooperation Strategy 2019–2023 provided a framework to guide the collective efforts of GMS countries in tackling health issues impacting the subregion. It had three strategic pillars:

- Strategic Pillar 1: Health security as a regional public good
- Strategic Pillar 2: Health impacts of connectivity and mobility
- Strategic Pillar 3: Health workforce development

Strategic Pillar 1 tackled the subregion's vulnerability to acute public health events. Strengthening mechanisms for multisector cooperation under the One Health approach was identified as a crucial building block for effective response to zoonotic diseases, AMR, and food safety threats. Under the strategy, "a One Health approach promotes the operational linking of sectors (public health, animal health, wildlife, environment, agriculture) to enable multistakeholder cooperation, information-sharing, and action for an effective response to health threats originating at the human–animal–ecosystems interface." Programming under this action area aimed to strengthen the foundation for One Health by integrating One Health principles in the projects of other GMS Program sectors. These included developing governance frameworks for the operational linking of health and non- health sectors, building animal health system capacity to align with that of public health systems, and harmonizing food safety systems.

The forthcoming GMS Health Cooperation Strategy 2024–2030 cites the transformational power of the One Health approach to advance intersectoral work in the GMS, not least because it is already well-understood by the countries of the GMS where it has been used for several years. Specifically, One Health is mentioned in the framework in relation to addressing AMR. This requires collaboration between animal and human health sectors on, for example, surveillance and research, appropriate use of antibiotics for both human and animal health, and effective sanitation, and infection prevention and control. One of the strategic pillars of the GMS Health Cooperation Strategy 2024–2030 is aimed at strengthening IHR capacities. The draft strategy also cites the transformational power of the One Health approach to advance intersectoral work in the GMS. The strategy will consider activities to improve AMR, including establishing a regional AMR surveillance network. The strategy could also provide opportunities to strengthen the existing One Health partnerships and networks in the region, for example the One Health Universities Network or the Consortium of Animal Market Networks to Assess Risk of Emerging Infectious Diseases through Enhanced Surveillance. The strategy's working group platform could serve to connect the efforts of these networks with the Regional Investment Framework and potential sources of funding from development partners.

Further Opportunities for One Health Action at ADB

In December 2023, ADB launched the Climate and Health Initiative (CHI) at the 28th United Nations Framework Convention on Climate Change Conference of the Parties (COP 28) as a key initiative under ADB's Climate Change Action Plan, 2023–2030. The CHI aims to strengthen climate and health policies and practices to deliver climate-resilient and low-carbon health care systems in ADB's DMCs and beyond through the six pillars of generating knowledge, mobilizing novel financing, forging partnerships, incubating innovations, building capacity, and championing advocacy. It will coordinate local, regional, and global climate-responsive health actions, grounded in a crosscutting One Health approach and its focus on low- and middle-income countries includes those in the GMS. Under the new GMS Health Cooperation Strategy 2024–2030, GMS countries are also exploring opportunities to strengthen their knowledge base in climate change and health, through a subregional platform and knowledge and financing partnerships.

ADB's new operating model, which came into effect in 2023, offers opportunities to advance work on One Health. The reorganization offers an opportunity to deliver integrated solutions through creation of multidisciplinary project teams, pulling staff together from across sectors, themes, and products, as needed. The One ADB approach should be applied when designing projects with One Health design, and good examples of this approach should be shared across the bank. The establishment of practice groups (for sectors and themes) at ADB, should prompt further collaboration on One Health nationally, across regional departments and through ADB's global interactions.

ADB's Asia Pacific Climate Finance Fund, a multi-donor trust fund established in April 2017, supports the development and implementation of financial risk management products that can help unlock capital for climate investments and improve resilience to the impact of climate change. One of its four financing priorities is promoting climate-sensitive sector investment, which explicitly includes agriculture, water and fisheries, areas with clear One Health overlap. This a good example of how One Health approaches can be incorporated into existing ADB operations and make the connection between One Health and climate change.

The forthcoming GMS Health Cooperation Strategy 2024–2030 cites the transformational power of the One Health approach to advance intersectoral work in the GMS, not least because it is already well-understood by the countries of the GMS where it has been used for several years.

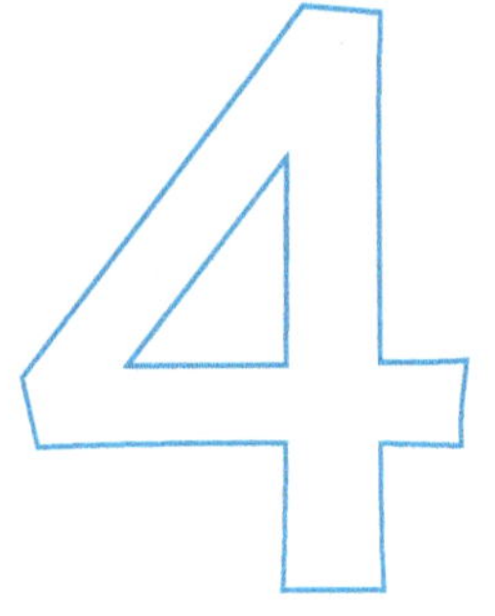 4 SCALING UP ONE HEALTH SOLUTIONS IN THE GREATER MEKONG SUBREGION

One Health approaches entail communication, coordination, collaboration, and integration across different sectors. While both national and regional One Health coordination efforts can be helpful as an important resource for countries, the One Health approach can be learned and implemented at all levels of government allowing for progress on managing locally important issues, often on a more accelerated timetable. Increased use of the One Health framework can happen simultaneously at all levels. Rather than wait for the creation of a regional coordinating body, it is better to have some short-term forward momentum on smaller scale initiatives while working toward a fully integrated One Health approach, as these can act as proof of concept in the GMS context, and provide invaluable data on cost vs. benefit.

National One Health Investment Examples

There are many One Health interventions that can be practically applied in the GMS context. Following are recommendations for country-driven One Health initiatives. These interventions are based on in-depth country consultations with GMS stakeholders and respond to the gaps and opportunities highlighted in Section 2: support One Health policy change

- strengthen surveillance
- reduce workforce constraints
- eliminate specific diseases (in this case rabies) and
- address climate change.

Invest in Policy: Analysis of Wildlife Trade Policy and Legislation to Improve Outcomes for Health Security and Biodiversity Conservation

Rationale

There is an urgent need to address use of wildlife in the GMS, both farmed and wild-caught, especially in wildlife use hot spots such as Cambodia, the Lao PDR, PRC, and Viet Nam. This is needed to reduce pandemic pathogen spillover risk and preserve biodiversity. Demands for bushmeat both domestically and for export remain high and encourage unethical and illegal harvest of wildlife. This demand contributes even further to pressure on wildlife populations harvested for trophies and for recovery of animal parts such as horns, tusks, skins, and other body parts, which have perceived value for ornamental purposes or in traditional medicine. Enhanced legislation and policies in this area are pivotal for tackling corruption, curbing transboundary movement and use of wildlife in the region, and importantly, minimizing human contact with zoonotic pathogens. By reducing wildlife trading, the threat of emerging infectious diseases and pandemics can be lowered. Actions in this area can also serve as a gateway to fortifying One Health policy and regulation on a broader scale, fostering cross-sectoral communication, and enhancing coordination among diverse stakeholders.

Practical Steps

- Review existing policies, legislation, and regulation, and revise it to include all species listed under the Convention on International Trade in Endangered Species of Wild Fauna and Flora.
- Collaborate with civil society organizations to engage the public in supporting law enforcement actions. Implement initiatives such as hotlines or reporting apps to facilitate public participation in reporting illegal wildlife activities.
- Legislate for interagency cooperation on intelligence and data sharing across national law enforcement agencies and between countries.
- Ensure appropriate resources and budget allocation to support law enforcement actions. Allocate funds for facilities dedicated to rescued wildlife and repatriation efforts, thereby preventing the reentry of these specimens into the illegal trade chain.
- Train enforcement and judiciary bodies, including joint training sessions on wildlife protection, bringing together prosecutors and judges.
- Have effective legislation criminalizing online wildlife sale and advertising.
- Take a harmonized approach to the regulation of trade in wildlife to minimize the existing inter-country disparities that make illegal behaviors worth the risk.

Invest in Surveillance: Integrating Wildlife Surveillance into National One Health Surveillance Systems

Rationale

Surveillance strategies play a critical role in pandemic preparedness, monitoring zoonotic diseases, combating AMR, and ensuring food safety, highlighting the importance of a One Health approach. Despite advancements in high-tech surveillance, basic zoonotic surveillance in the region requires improvement. Urgent action is needed to enhance AMR surveillance due to limited resources and scarce baseline data. Global plans and protocols endorsed by WHO address AMR, emphasizing the interconnectedness of human, animal, plant, and environmental health.

Food safety surveillance should consider the role of animals in the food production chain, focusing on preharvest, postharvest, and retail phases. Challenges in the GMS, like fragmented food systems and inadequate surveillance, must be addressed. Environmental surveillance, within a One Health framework, demands careful planning considering livestock practices, environmental management, mining, and forestry.

Utilizing advanced surveillance approaches, including predictive modeling, is essential to tackle the complexity of sampling strategies. While One Health approaches promise improved intervention effectiveness and cost savings, a systematic assessment of their impact on surveillance is lacking. Anticipated benefits include enhanced efficiency and cost-effectiveness, though country-specific contexts must be considered. ADB, with expertise in financial analysis, is well-positioned to contribute to evaluating the economic value of One Health-integrated surveillance.

Practical Steps

- Share resources more equitably between human, wildlife, and environmental health services. Provide domestic or international funding that requires clear collaboration and equitable decision-making power between human health, animal health, and other stakeholders.
- Implement the wildlife health surveillance systems developed in several GMS countries at a national scale, and link these to disease surveillance systems in other sectors.
- Legislate for data sharing across human health, animal health, and environment sector stakeholders at all levels, to promote data systems interoperability.
- Standardize One Health data indicators and reporting requirements across institutions.
- Allocate sufficient resources to improve diagnostic facilities and sample collection and enhance collaboration between private and public sector laboratories.

Build the Capacity of the Workforce in the Animal Health and Environment Sectors

Rationale

Throughout the GMS, there is an imbalance of workforce capacity in between the human health, and animal health and environment sector. This hampers zoonotic disease prevention at the source and prevents implementation of risk-based prevention of unknown disease threats, due to weak surveillance systems.

Workforce strengthening can reduce the disease burden in human populations through control of animal reservoirs and/or more rapid detection of potential outbreaks; improve agricultural and rural livelihoods through better control of endemic diseases and addressing livestock/agricultural production constraints; and reduce inappropriate use of antimicrobials in the animal health sector.

A widespread problem in the region is the lack of understanding of epidemiological principles for planning and conducting surveillance. The region also requires comprehensive epidemiology training and both basic and advanced levels.

More efforts are needed to ensure that the animal and environmental sectors can meet a minimum standard of performance before placing overly high expectations on their contribution to One Health efforts.

Practical Steps

- Assess the size, type, distribution, and level of training of the animal health and environmental workforce.
- Create a national workforce strategy for the recruitment, retention, and professional development of veterinarians, para-veterinarians, environmental scientists, ecologists, wildlife rangers and other related professions.

- Provide monetary and political support to improve workforce capabilities, to ensure they have the required resources, transportation, and communication tools to effectively conduct their roles.

Invest in Disease-Specific Initiatives: Accelerated Regional Rabies Elimination

Rationale

Rabies is a deadly disease that results in the deaths of an estimated 59,000 people each year, and tens of thousands more animals.[67] There is a human vaccine for rabies but the most cost-effective and efficient means to eliminate it in both humans and domestic dogs is to vaccinate the domestic dog population, an approach already adopted in many countries. This has led to major economic and health benefits. It provides a compelling example of how to prevent human rabies deaths, but in the process also shows how to strengthen One Health capacity for other endemic and emerging infectious diseases. It is also timely—the ASEAN regional strategy to eliminate rabies is currently being updated to align with the 2030 global rabies elimination goal.

Rabies control brings reduced expenditure in the human health sector for reactive provision of human post-exposure prophylaxis, and resources can be reallocated to the animal health sector for dog vaccination. Overall, there should be economic and health benefits through reduced overall rabies expenditure. A strong rabies detection system also contributes to a broader system for the early detection and prevention of other zoonotic disease spillover events (including potential pandemics).

Practical Steps

- Allocate resources for full implementation of national and regional rabies elimination plans.
- Scale up vaccine and medicines banks (including canine rabies vaccine, human post-exposure prophylaxis vaccines, and rabies immunoglobulin).
- Increase opportunities for bilateral and regional knowledge and resource sharing.
- Provide funding for operational research targeted at identifying optimal strategies for mass dog vaccination to reduce canine rabies transmission.
- Implement integrated rabies surveillance and response at national level.
- Reduce costs of providing post-exposure prophylaxis.
- Increase awareness and behavior change to reduce rabies exposure risks.

Enhance Climate Change Adaptation Through Nature Conservation

Rationale

The relationship between investments in One Health and in climate change response is two-way. Investments to adapt to climate change and mitigate against its impact can have diverse benefits that cut across human, animal, and agricultural sectors. These include reduced risk of pandemics through decreased risk of zoonotic spillover, greater protection from natural disasters, improved water quality, and even increased tourism opportunities. In the other direction, One Health investments can yield an innate climate change dividend. Conserving,

---

[67] World Health Organization. Rabies.

sustainably managing, and restoring natural habitats provide a significant and cost-effective contribution to tackling climate change. In particular, tropical rainforests are important ecosystems for mitigating climate change. Tropical rainforests collectively sequester more carbon from the atmosphere than temperate or boreal forest. Conservation of natural habitats is also critical for addressing the major issue of global biodiversity loss, and the GMS is a biodiversity hot spot.

Practical Steps

- Improve monitoring of the illegal wildlife trade.
- Provide incentives for the conservation of natural habitats and implement measures to reduce the illegal timber trade.
- Support sustainable intensification of agricultural production. Actions such as improving agricultural extension, improving market linkages, reducing harvest and consumption waste can reduce the pressure on expanding agricultural land into natural habitats.

Regional One Health Investment Examples

Working Together for One Health

Because One Health actions are complex, and cut across multiple sectors they demand extra coordination, both among development partners and within governments. Joint action and coordination among key development partners is critical to successful One Health programming. This applies to partners with a diverse range of mandates, including human and animal health, environmental protection, gender, development finance and climate change.

It will be essential to complement this arrangement with standards and guidance, technical tools and training, advice on use of economic and costing analysis tools, and assistance with information technology tools and applications. This is where technical agencies like World Organization for Animal Health (WOAH), WHO, UNEP, and FAO will come into their own. These agencies have a comparative advantage in addressing zoonoses, and other health risks at the human–animal–ecosystem interface, in particular in terms of norms and guidance, while the multilateral development banks are in a position to provide the necessary financing and TA.

The WHO South-East Asia Regional Office (SEARO) has recently accepted responsibilities of the Quadripartite Secretariat from 2023 to 2025. To facilitate planning during the SEARO Secretariat term, the Asia Pacific Quadripartite organized the First Asia Pacific Quadripartite One Health Workshop from 5–8 September 2023 in Bangkok, Thailand. The main objectives of the workshop were to advocate and familiarize attendees with the Quadripartite One Health Joint Plan of Action[68] and its Implementation Guide,[69] support member states to better understand and adapt the Joint Plan of Action to their national context, and raise awareness of One Health issues across the human–animal–plant and wider environment interface to the official representatives of the member states and other international partners organizations.

---

[68] Food and Agriculture Organization of the United Nations, UN Environment Programme, World Health Organization, World Organisation for Animal Health. One Health Joint Plan of Action (2022–2026). Working Together for the Health of Humans, Animals, Plants and the Environment. 2022.

[69] The Food and Agriculture Organization of the United Nations, United Nations Environment Programme, the World Health Organization, and World Organisation for Animal Health. 2023. *A Guide to Implementing the One Health Joint Plan of Action at National Level.* Geneva.

Establishing a Regional Coordination Body

GMS countries remain committed to have in place national action plans on health security, AMR, food safety, or One Health. Countries lacking specific action plans are exposed and likely to be more vulnerable in case of a new outbreak. Revision of existing national action plans to incorporate lessons from events like the COVID-19 pandemic and evaluations such as the Joint External Evaluation or Performance of Veterinary Services is essential. At the national level, efforts should persist in developing governance frameworks that operationally link health and non-health sectors.

To prevent future outbreaks, GMS countries should also invest in expanding scientific research on zoonoses, regulate and monitor traditional food markets, incentivize legal wildlife trade and animal husbandry with zoonotic control measures, and radically transform food systems. These areas are pivotal for informed strategies and policy responses to safeguard against future health crises.

Some GMS public health emergency capabilities are best built at a national level, but others are best addressed subregionally or regionally (Table 4). As health security in the GMS is influenced by both country-specific and regional collective actions, stronger mechanisms for multisector One Health cooperation are essential.

Virtually no country in the world has a fully self-sufficient food supply and foods of animal origin are a known risk for the occurrence of zoonotic diseases in humans. Therefore, import and export of safe food should logically be part of any regional One Health initiative as maintaining a robust supply chain of safe food would contribute to a country's resilience against future pandemics. For example, existing working groups on agriculture and health could join forces and collaborate to address issues of mutual concern related to biosecurity and public health. Taking a One Health approach to enhance the capacity for safe and traceable intraregional food supply would contribute significantly to food security. This would not only enhance a country's resilience against future pandemics but would also acknowledge the limited self-sufficiency of any nation in terms of food supply. Similarly, although countries should implement comprehensive measures to control distribution and use of antimicrobials within their borders, this will not completely manage AMR in a country. AMR has its own transmission pathways that are related not only to non-judicious use of antimicrobials in humans and animals, but also to cross-border AMR vectors associated with the environment (fresh or marine water, effluent) and trade of animals and animal products. Therefore, a regional perspective is crucial for comprehensive AMR management.

Issues pertaining to One Health in relation to wildlife, including waterfowl, inherently transcend national borders due to practical constraints on confining or excluding these species within a specific country. While regional planning plays a pivotal role in managing the legal trade of wildlife and its products, it also serves as a catalyst for heightened awareness and improved management strategies concerning wildlife and bird migration. Recognizing the interconnected nature of these challenges underscores the importance of collaborative, cross-border efforts in addressing One Health concerns associated with wildlife and bird populations. Such regional initiatives not only facilitate effective wildlife management but also foster a broader understanding of the ecological complexities inherent in the movement of these species across geopolitical boundaries.

Given the wealth of expertise in the UN Quadripartite One Health High-Level Expert Panel, an excellent reference point for future joint action in the GMS is the global consensus on One Health priorities, laid out in a 2023 UN Quadripartite call to action for One Health for a safer world.[70] The Quadripartite urged all countries and key takeholders to promote seven priority actions (Box 6).

---

[70]   World Health Organization. 2023. Quadripartite call to action for One Health for a safer world. Press Release. 27 March.

TABLE 4 Public Health Emergency Capabilities Better-Suited to Be Built at the Regional or Subregional Level

Regional Opportunity	Function	National Dependencies
Cross-border collaboration	Build and maintain, collaboration and coordination among border points of entry and in all relevant sectors	Harmonized border procedures, legal basis for cross-border data sharing, professional cross-border peer groups, cross-ministerial One Health committees
Field epidemiology	Standardize field epidemiology training across countries Set up train the trainer programs	Sufficient human resources, retention of trained staff; epidemiology and One Health integrated into medical and veterinary curricula; spatial database of farms and livestock
Incident management systems	Promote transparency and real-time data sharing through standardized operating procedures and training	National action plans for zoonosis, One Health, antimicrobial resistance. Clear guidance on areas of responsibility for surveillance and response in a health emergency
Medical countermeasures	Support regional level approvals, manufacturing sourcing and distribution of medicines during an emergency	Medicines, vaccines, and personal protective equipment stockpiling;
Surge capacity	Help countries establish human resources reserves before they are needed	Diagnostic testing capacity and load-balancing strategy; ability to utilize veterinary laboratories for processing human samples (and vice-versa)
Information technology	Use advanced data analytics on large data sets to monitor and respond to public health emergencies	Legal basis to share information between sectors and laboratory systems, digital data capture in interoperable databases, good data warehousing, data management training and compliance

Source: McKinsey & Company.

BOX 6

United Nations Quadripartite Organizations Call to Action for One Health for a Safer World

Stressing the need for enhanced collaboration and commitment to translate the One Health approach into policy action in all countries, the Quadripartite leaders urge all countries and key stakeholders to promote and undertake the following priority actions.

1. Prioritize One Health in the international political agenda, increase understanding and advocate for the adoption and promotion of the enhanced intersectoral health governance. The One Health approach should notably serve as a guiding principle in global mechanisms; including in the new pandemic instrument and the Pandemic Fund to strengthen pandemic prevention, preparedness and response;

2. Strengthen national One Health policies, strategies and plans, costed and prioritized in line with the Quadripartite One Health Joint Plan of Action, to foster wider implementation across relevant sectors and at all levels;

3. Accelerate the implementation of One Health plans, including supporting of national One Health governance and multisectoral coordination mechanisms, development of situation analyses, stakeholder mapping, priority setting, and metrics for One Health monitoring and evaluation frameworks;

4. Build intersectoral One Health work forces that have the skills, capacities, and capabilities to prevent, detect, control, and respond to health threats in a timely and effective way, by strengthening joint pre-service and continuing education for human, animal, and environmental health work forces;

5. Strengthen and sustain prevention of pandemics and health threats at source, targeting activities and places that increase the risk of zoonotic spillover between animals to humans;

6. Encourage and strengthen One Health scientific knowledge and evidence creation and exchange, research and development, technology transfer and sharing and integrating of information and data and facilitate access to new tools and technologies; and

7. Increase investment and financing of One Health strategies and plans ensuring scaled up implementation at all levels, including funding for prevention of health threats at source.

Source: World Health Organization. 2023. Call to Action for One Health for a Safer World.

Given the global interdependence on food supplies, countries should include import and export of safe food as integral components of regional One Health initiatives.

Priority Recommendations to Accelerate One Health Action in the Greater Mekong Subregion

These recommendations are aligned with the UN Quadripartite call to action priority actions and respond to regional gaps.

1.   **Build on existing One Health coordination mechanisms.** There are three existing platforms for One Health coordination in the region: the UN One Health Quadripartite, the ASEAN One Health Network, and the GMS Working Group for Health Cooperation. All three organizations have a strong mandate on One Health and are therefore in a unique position to jointly and individually demonstrate scale up of One Health across the region. This work is underpinned by the APHSAF framework. One Health coordination mechanisms exist in several GMS countries, but existing One Health activities should be expanded from intersectoral discussions to practical actions to address clearly defined One Health issues. In particular, there is a need for greater collaboration with the environment sector, which has been somewhat neglected relative to the human and animal health sectors in the evolution of One Health. This can be done by enhancing the existing or planned governance and coordination structures to actively include the sector. Supporting one strategy, one coordination mechanism and one monitoring system on One Health under the government's leadership is key for a sustainable response.

2.   **Invest in institutional capacity and coordination.** Capacity and coordination improvements are needed across human health, animal health, wildlife, and environment sectors. This is common to the six GMS countries, but each will have its own focus areas, such as workforce strengthening, infrastructure, resourcing, or data management. COVID-19 showed the importance of investing in laboratory operations, cold chains, community engagement, and disease tracing and data management. Identifying sustainable financing will require increased advocacy to higher levels of government for domestic One Health funding. Developing pilot projects to demonstrate the practical benefits of One Health to local communities can help make the business case. More training and research is also required—this can be achieved through partnerships with universities, communities, and the private sector.

3.   **Seek out opportunities for regional collaboration to share the cost burden and learn from others.** The new GMS Health Cooperation Strategy emphasizes the key role of regional cooperation and integration to collectively address transnational challenges. Better data sharing across sectors would support more effective One Health planning and preparedness. This is especially important in Cambodia, the Lao PDR, and Myanmar, but increased cross-sectoral system interoperability will benefit all parts of the GMS. One mechanism to bolster regional One Health collaboration would be to work through the new ASEAN Centre for Public Health Emergencies and Emerging Diseases, though other types of cooperative agreements should also be considered for very specific One Health sectors such as agri-food production and AMR, as discussed in the previous section.